The Practices of
Yoga for the
Digestive System

Dr Swami Shankardevananda
MBBS (Sydney), MSc (UNSW)

Under the Guidance of
Swami Satyananda Saraswati

Yoga Publications Trust, Munger, Bihar, India

Published by Bihar School of Yoga
    First edition 1979
    Reprinted 1980
    Second edition 1987
    Reprinted 1993

Published by Yoga Publications Trust
    Third edition 2003
    Reprinted 2005, 2008, 2009

ISBN: 978-81-85787-25-1

Publisher and distributor: Yoga Publications Trust, Ganga Darshan, Munger, Bihar, India.

Website: www.biharyoga.net
          www.rikhiapeeth.net

Printed at Thomson Press (India) Limited, New Delhi, 110001

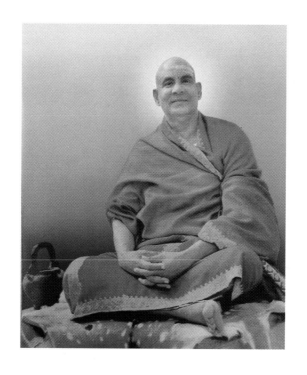

Dedication

In humility we offer this dedication to
Swami Sivananda Saraswati, who initiated
Swami Satyananda Saraswati into the secrets of yoga.

Contents

Practical Digestion

Appendices

Preface

The digestive tract is one of the great paradoxes of life. On the one hand it lies within our bodies, controlled by the unconscious aspects of the mind and autonomic nervous system. On the other hand, most people do not realize just how much of their waking lives is concerned with this unknown entity; how much of their time is consumed in the various food-related activities of buying, preparing and eating three or more meals each day.

Hunger comes; we become aware of the gnawing feeling, though we are not always fully aware of what is really happening inside; then we satisfy our need. Some time later we feel the urge to empty our bowels, so once again the digestive tract comes into the field of our awareness. What happens in between these times is a mystery of the workings of the body. Things just seem to happen inside and they do not really need our conscious attention, or do they? Occasionally the thought does come into our awareness as to what does go on inside this box we call the body.

Even during times when we become aware of our digestive process, we are not fully conscious or able to have complete conscious understanding of the body's workings. For most of us, activity concerned with the digestive tract is habitual, routine, repetitive and subconscious. We rarely enjoy food with the gusto of one eating for the first time and we are taught to regard defecation as anything but pleasurable.

King Akbar was enjoying a great feast as he sat on a bed of cushions, entertained by beautiful dancing girls.

"What is the most enjoyable pleasure in the whole world?" he asked Birbal, his cleverest minister.

Birbal replied, "Going to the toilet."

"What! You mean to say you enjoy sitting on the toilet more than all this beautiful food and all these beautiful dancing. girls?"

Birbal replied, "Without a doubt, your Majesty, going to the toilet is one of my greatest pleasures."

Everyone laughed at his reply, and so Birbal, determined to prove his point, made a plan. The next evening, as Akbar was being entertained, he put a potent laxative into the king's wine. The laxative quickly took effect and a short time later the king felt a pressing need to relieve his bowels. Just as he started to get up, Birbal ordered one of the king's most beautiful girls to perform his favourite dance, so the king was forced to sit, torn between his two desires.

"I must leave you for a moment, Birbal," he said, once more starting to rise.

"But Your Majesty," Birbal protested, "they are just bringing out your favourite meal. Don't you think you should eat it while it is hot?"

Again the king sat down, this time looking a little worried, for the inner pressure was building up slowly but surely. At last, with one mouthful of his favourite food still in his mouth, the king stood up quickly and ran out of the room. A little while later he came back, a big smile on his face.

"You were right, Birbal. There is nothing more pleasurable than that."

The digestive system can be the doorway to some of our most enjoyable moments and, if we treat it sensibly, to dynamic, vital health. Using yoga we can extend the basic functions of the digestive process so as to gain even more pleasure and fulfilment in life, for yoga allows us to become fully aware of the unconscious aspects of digestion. This is a part of the awakening of manipura chakra and results in an incredible injection of power, vitality and dynamism into our lives.

Many people claim to have perfect digestion. However, even these people can improve the quality of their conscious control over the digestive tract and thereby are better able to tap the vast source of energy and good health within the natural processes of the body. The hatha yoga shatkarmas (cleansing techniques), for example, open the door to the immense treasure of energy that remains dormant within each human being.

It is our aim in this book to help open the doorway to the digestive process to all. The first step in the awakening of our dormant power is to gain access to the knowledge of the inner workings of the body and the mind. This is found in the first part of the book (The Digestive Process). Then we must know what can go wrong with the delicate, sensitive but resilient machinery, in the form of disease, as found in part two (Digestive Disorders). Equipped with this theoretical knowledge plus the practical techniques of yoga, we can begin to remove the first layer of dirt and impurities which cloud our health in the form of disease. Then we can begin to relax the inner tension until eventually a point is reached when an explosion of awareness and energy takes place.

This book has been written from personal experience, under the training of our guru, Swami Satyananda Saraswati. In becoming able to deal with the yogic lifestyle, each person in this ashram has had to totally re-evaluate their understanding of life. To achieve anything in yoga we must start with the basics, and diet and food are amongst the most essential aspects of our survival. Only when we have gone through the first layer of needs, desires, instincts and intuitions, can we start to really live yoga from moment to moment, opening the doorway to the higher life at the physical, emotional, mental, psychic and spiritual levels.

Swami Satyananda's approach to diet is pure and simple and is the basis of all the material in this book. Most people who attempt to follow the ashram diet, find that there is always some difficulty in adjusting from a more complicated western diet or the richer, spicier and heavier Indian diet. Occasionally, diarrhoea may occur, or indigestion, or severe and unremitting craving may drive some desperate soul to the local market in an attempt to drown his internal suffering with his favourite food. Whatever the obstacle that comes up, there is a method by which it can be surmounted, and that is by maintaining awareness and a positive attitude.

Whenever an ashramite gets a bout of ashram diarrhoea, it is not looked upon as being a disease process but as a cleansing one. All the malfunctions are traced back to the origin within the mind; and on the way we observe the mental scenery. Many cravings arise; hunger may be absent at one time and later we may be ravenous; tastes change; the senses become sharpened; our conscious appreciation of food deepens; our realization of the place of food in our lives is put into perspective with all the other phases of existence. All the so-called problems of life become transformed into the means of expanding our consciousness.

It is our hope that after you have read this book and have started to apply it in your life, your digestion, in all its phases, will become one of the great pleasures in your life.

The Digestive Process

1

Introduction

Indigestion is everyone's problem. Regardless of whether we are suffering from a digestive problem at the moment or not, each one of us suffers from indigestion in any of its many forms at some time or other. For most people it is not possible to predict when or how the next bout will come, but that it will come some time is inevitable. This common problem, which has such adverse effects on our whole mental outlook and our ability to function efficiently and joyously, certainly deserves more understanding and effective treatment than it has been receiving up to now.

Indigestion is actually a deeper problem than most of us realize. In order to understand this condition completely we must examine it from all angles and depths. On the surface we see it as being caused by chronic overeating or bad eating habits but, beneath the surface, mental tensions and negative attitudes which direct us towards debilitating habits are perhaps the most important factors. Working at unconscious levels, these basic seed problems sprout and grow in the digestive tract and spread from there into other systems of the body.

Anger, tension and frustration lower our functional efficiency level. Eating in these states either makes us physically sick through dyspepsia and other conditions or mentally frustrated through lack of satisfaction and enjoyment. Thus work suffers, family life and relationships suffer. At the cellular level the body mistimes the various processes because of lack of adequate nervous and endocrine control. When the body's controls break down we become prone to disease. The digestive system, being the most sensitive in many people, is the first to become upset and the stomach voices the complaint.

Digestive problems are a sign of impending danger, not just at the physical level, but at social and economic levels as well. Poor digestion caused by stresses and bad living and eating habits plays a large role in the turmoil and chaos of the world today. One can well imagine what is subconsciously influencing the minds of politicians, businessmen and women and top level executives when at some important meeting, perhaps to decide long-term policy, a stomach ulcer or painful haemorrhoid begins to play up. How can people in positions of responsibility make correct decisions under constant pressure from external sources while at the same time suffering from the strain of a weak digestive tract? Surely many executives are desperate to find permanent relief from these constantly recurring and greatly distressing problems.

Digestive upsets, particularly peptic ulcers, account for a vast loss of working hours, resulting in decreased economic productivity. At the individual level they result in suffering and the inability to live active, satisfying and full lives The obese person is a prime example of one who suffers tremendously from an inability to function efficiently.

Indigestion may not appear to be as catastrophic as some of the disasters and crises facing humankind today. It lacks the impact and dramatic quality of cyclones, drought, war, etc. However, the present state of world-wide indigestion is more insidious than the gross, short-lived, acute catastrophes which make headlines. Indigestion is a serious threat to productive living, not in itself but in the fact that it seems like such a small and simple disorder in our complicated lives that we tend to neglect it. As a result it becomes chronic and eventually saps our strength, vigour and vitality. We feel run down due to poor assimilation of

4

food, but do not realize the link between the loss of energy and indigestion. In this slow process we are actually letting our vital reserves leak away the longer we refuse to acknowledge and repair our faulty digestion. Then, because there is no reserve of good heath and resistance, any slight imbalance or stress can tip the scales precipitating us into the disease state.

This complex interplay of emotional and physical states which leads to indigestion has been thoroughly investigated by yoga and allied sciences. Yoga is now internationally recognized as a powerful means to balance both bodily systems and alleviate the stormy passions of the mind which lead to digestive upset. It quells the disturbances which lead to both inner and outer turmoil in the form of dyspepsia, diarrhoea, etc. as well as conflicting interrelationships. Instead of using purgatives, antacids and other harmful chemical substances which sap our strength, willpower and ability to control inner body processes, yoga offers a way to tackle the problems of the mind that lead concomitantly to digestive upset and external chaos.

A combination of yoga and other sciences aimed at rebalancing the basic disequilibrium of the body may be the answer to many of our digestive problems. The potential combination of yoga and allopathy should be examined carefully by all members of the healing profession. To many doctors, yoga may seem to be opposed to traditional medical science. From our experience, however, nothing could be further from the truth. Even if yoga proves to be a panacea for all illnesses, there are few people in the world who could utilize it in all situations, especially in the acute or serious disease situation. More than likely, yoga will initially emerge as a powerful adjunct to medical science. Just as doctors now utilize other specialities when they reach the limits of their own field of competence, so yoga can be used. Those people, for example, who prefer the medical means of therapy for the acute stages of digestive illness can utilize yogic techniques during convalescence when drugs have been withdrawn. In the troublesome field of chronic psychosomatic and degenerative disease, the combination of yoga and medicine may prove to be the answer that many doctors and patients are looking for.

At present medical science alone is unable to cure many digestive disorders because of the underlying mental factor that is involved. Powerful techniques are required to release the mental problems and purify the body. The science of yoga has developed such techniques over thousands of years, so it is really not necessary to view peptic ulcer, constipation and other forms of indigestion as lifetime diseases. A few weeks of yoga therapy, preferably in the ashram environment, is generally all that is required to initiate a complete reversal in the disease process and to eliminate unpleasant symptoms.

From our experience at the Bihar School of Yoga, managing a wide variety of disease conditions from arthritis to cancer, we have found that the digestive system plays an important role. Not only have we seen that indigestion and poor eating habits play a primary role in body breakdown and serious chronic disease, but that through the digestive tract we can effectively treat many conditions, for example, asthma. The digestive system running down the centre of the body seems to be the key to good health, in terms of its physical proximity to many organs, its powerful link with the mind and its physiological connection with manipura chakra, the centre of energy and physical health.

The demand for yogic techniques to remedy various digestive problems has become so great that our guru, Swami Satyananda Saraswati, inspired this work in order to help people combat indigestion and end the vicious circle of spiralling bad health. To ascertain the scope of this huge and up to now uncorrelated subject, we have had to rely on the teachings of our guru and on yogic scriptures as well as modern and ancient medical texts. Allopathy, ayurveda, acupuncture and modern psychology have all been researched to complete the picture.

By utilizing the theoretical and practical knowledge contained here, you will gain a deeper understanding of the structure and function of the digestive tract and how it is affected by diet and lifestyle. In this way a sensible, positive and creative approach towards food and eating in all its aspects can be developed. This will automatically lead to increased awareness of the digestive process and control over what is ingested. As one's life becomes more natural and simple, the body and mind are simultaneously harmonized and the cloud of indigestion passes to reveal the light of good health, dynamism and sublime equanimity.

2

The Digestive System

Because many people today are suffering from digestive disorders of one sort or another, a basic understanding of the digestive system is important in the quest for better health. For those interested in spiritual development an awareness of the digestive processes will be an aid to the attainment of physical and mental balance. This alone can lead to peace and well being, for mind and body work together as one unit to form one being. What helps the body helps the mind, and vice versa. Awareness of the body is part of a traditional meditative practice. Knowledge of the anatomy and physiology of the body is a big help in giving our bodily awareness form and substance. This can then manifest in our everyday life as awareness of bodily functions and needs which, when satisfied, lead to good health.

The digestive system consists of approximately 32 feet of tubing that starts at the mouth and ends at the anus. The tract is a special system concerned with the transport and assimilation of foods and fluids, and the rejection of undigested particles, plus other waste matter from the body.

The process of digestion occurs in consecutive stages, one blending into the other with no clear subdivisions. The following is a basic classification that is useful in terms of understanding the processes:

1. *Ingestion*: Food is taken into the digestive canal through the mouth, pharynx and oesophagus.

2. *Secretion and digestion*: Enzymes, acids and other chemicals are secreted for the breakdown of food into smaller particles. This process starts in the mouth and continues into the small intestine.
3. *Absorption*: Water and small soluble units, the breakdown products of digestion, are absorbed in the small intestine mainly and to a lesser extent in the large intestine.
4. *Assimilation*: Food that has been absorbed is transported via the bloodstream and utilized by the cells of the body.
5. *Rejection*: Undigested particles of food are expelled from the rectum and anus. This process also removes poisons from the body and is part of the general process of cleaning and assimilation that goes on continually.

The fate of each mouthful

The digestive tract is a hollow tube uninterrupted in its continuity, except for odd valves interspersed between the many sections. The only way food can reach the cells is to be assimilated and absorbed, which requires the complex process described above. Try to visualize in yourself this structure passing from end to end, like a tube, with the rest of the body wrapped around it.

When food particles are ingested they must be digested, absorbed and assimilated. This transformation is aided by secretions of the mouth, stomach, liver, gall bladder and pancreas. The whole process goes on continually, without a break, until all the food ingested is assimilated and all the wastes are disposed of.

The process is thus a smooth flowing continuum and each part is dependent on the other parts for its efficient functioning. If one step goes wrong the whole process is disturbed and a vicious circle of bad health results. For example, when the digestive juices are not flowing in a balanced and regulated manner, then assimilation and absorption cannot take place. The whole organism is so integrated and dependent on its parts that if one part is not working the whole body suffers.

Food enters the mouth and the process begins, triggered by the sensory mechanism of seeing the food prepared and ready to eat. If the food looks unappetizing, or if the body is not hungry, then the mind and brain do not trigger the digestive juices to function. Therefore, eat when you are hungry that food which is appetizing and good for you.

Within the mouth, the teeth, palate, tongue and salivary glands all function together to make the food into a bolus, which will travel neatly into the stomach. It is important at this stage to chew your food well so that it can be digested more easily.

The taste buds are essential for the process of digestion. Not only do they ensure the correct secretion of digestive juices in the mouth, they tell us if the food is health-giving or not and through them the taste experience is transmitted to the mind thus begetting mental satisfaction. Once the food passes from the mouth it is usually forgotten, unless we cultivate yogic awareness and try to follow it through the many different channels of the body. This can be a very rewarding pastime.

Food passes down the oesophagus, which secretes a lubricant to aid the passage of food into the stomach. The swallowing process is quite complex and involves the movement of the tongue to throw the food into the oesophagus, so cutting off the air passages. This prevents food from passing into the lungs, which is a very uncomfortable sensation. Next time you swallow, close your eyes and try to follow the movement. Become aware of exactly what happens in this common but usually unconscious process.

In the stomach the food is churned and digested by the acids and enzymes secreted by the stomach wall. There are two types of stomach movement occurring during digestion:
1. In the stomach wall, muscles exert a steady and slight pressure which squeezes the food downwards towards the pylorus. This movement pushes the food stored in the upper part of the stomach towards the lower end where it enters the small intestine.

10

The Digestive System

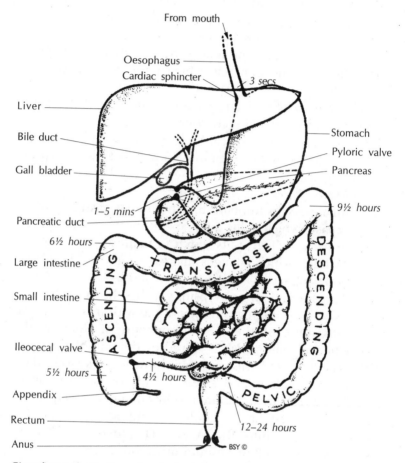

Given figures denote time taken for first particles of food eaten to reach that point

2. A vigorous contracting movement mixes and churns the food with digestive juices and pushes it into the first part of the small intestine. The gastric juices include hydrochloric acid and enzymes such as pepsin, lipase and rennin (to break down milk protein and fats). The stomach secretes hormones whose exact functions are still not fully known, such as gastrin. It also secretes

mucin, which forms a barrier to keep the stomach from digesting itself and prevents ulcers forming on the wall of the stomach. Acid and mucin secretion must be balanced for proper digestion.

In the duodenum the food is further digested by juices from the liver and pancreas which pour down a common duct (tube).

The pancreas is a large gland which lies behind the stomach and gives two secretions:

1. *Insulin*, which pours into the bloodstream and helps the blood glucose to be taken into body cells after absorption takes place.

2. *Pancreatic juices* which contain:
   a) Alkaline salts to neutralize the potent gastric acids
   b) Lipase, which splits fats
   c) Amylase, which splits starch to maltose
   d) Maltase, which changes maltose to glucose (the basic body sugar)
   e) Trypsin and chymotrypsin, which split protein

The liver is a highly complex organ with many different functions. One of the most important of these is the production of bile, which is stored in the gall bladder just under the liver. It is this compound which gives faeces their characteristic colour and smell. It aids the absorption of fats, cholesterol (an important product in the correct quantity but not in excess) and vitamins D and K. The liver also stores iron, vitamins B_{12}, A and D, glucose for use in emergencies, as well as fats and other substances.

The liver breaks down or detoxifies many of the poisons and chemicals entering and made by the body. It is concerned with destruction of red blood cells as well as the manufacture of protein and other important substances. The liver purifies our blood and maintains the body processes. It is such an important organ that we cannot do without it.

After leaving the duodenum, food passes into the jejunum, another part of the small intestine. This tube of muscle (over 20 feet long) called the 'small' intestine is not

12

really small, but it is usually thinner than the large intestine, which is shorter. Food is continually being digested and passed down the intestines. A continual churning motion allows all of the food to come into contact with the muscle wall, where absorption takes place of substances such as amino acids (proteins), sugars, minerals, glycerol, fats, vitamins and glycerides. Capillaries and lacteals are the structures designed to absorb these different substances and transport them into the main part of the bloodstream for distribution to the whole body. It is the cells of the wall that actually do the work of carrying digested food products into the blood.

The large intestine is approximately six feet long. Its function is to absorb water and salts into the blood so that the body does not lose too much of these valuable substances. By drying out faeces we retain the fluids and salts and allow stool to form. Mucus is secreted by the muscle walls and this neutralizes and lubricates the faeces, acting also as a barrier and defence against bacteria.

The sigmoid colon, part of the large intestine, stores the faeces until there is enough to stimulate the desire to defecate.

Faeces are mainly the residue from the small intestine and contain:

1. Residues of indigestible material in food, such as the skins of fruit and vegetables (mainly cellulose)
2. Bile
3. Intestinal secretions, including mucus
4. White blood cells
5. Cells from the walls of the intestine
6. Numerous bacteria, which make up one third of the total solids
7. Inorganic material (10–20%)

Note that very little digestible material is present.

Defecation is a complex reflex act. As the passage of faeces into the rectum distends the muscular tube, signals are sent to the conscious and unconscious parts of the brain. This brings about a conscious voluntary decision to inhibit or permit reflex evacuation. If we are relaxed, the process occurs all the more efficiently. The parasympathetic system, which is concerned with the relaxation of the whole body, allows the sphincters to open and the muscle wall to contract, propelling faeces out of the anus. It is important not to strain on the toilet because this stimulates the sympathetic system which closes the sphincters all the more tightly. The only healthy way to defecate is with a relaxed mind.

After swallowing

Food takes approximately three seconds to travel from the mouth to the stomach. It takes one to five minutes for the first mouthful to enter the duodenum and 20 minutes for half the consumed food to leave the stomach. In 4½ hours the first mouthful has reached the start of the large intestine, the caecum. The first mouthful of food takes 9½ hours to reach the end of the large intestine, the sigmoid colon. From start to finish the complete process of digestion takes from 12 to 24 hours.

Next time you have a meal, try to increase your body awareness by following the process of digestion in your body. You will have to remember throughout the day that the process is going on and make an effort to increase your awareness. This can be practised anytime and anywhere. There should be no limitations to your awareness and no mental blocks or complexes concerning bodily functions.

The three main centres

1. The mouth: The process of digestion really starts in the mouth. The salivary glands constantly secrete saliva at the rate of half a gallon per day. Saliva contains the enzyme ptylin, which breaks down starch. Chewing mixes saliva into the food, which tends to neutralize stomach acids to a certain extent.

2. The stomach: This organ is about the size of your hands cupped together. To fill the stomach we need eat no more than this quantity. However, the stomach can stretch

14

to enormous proportions to accommodate the sometimes enormous amounts of food we deposit in it. For optimal digestion fill the stomach with one-third solid, one-third liquid and one-third air.

Food stays in the stomach for two to six hours, depending on the type of food consumed. Fats and meat are harder to digest than lighter food such as carbohydrates. This is why a light vegetarian meal gives more energy and does not create a feeling of fullness or heaviness. When we eat a big meal more blood is drained from the brain and other vital organs to the stomach for greater periods of time than a light small meal, and thus we may feel sleepy after a large meal.

3. The intestines: The inside of the small intestine feels like velvet. The wall contains hundreds of thousands of microscopic villi (hair-like nodules) which contain the blood vessels and lacteals to absorb nutrients. The large numbers of villi increase the surface area enormously. It is estimated that the absorbing surface area of the small intestine is 75,000 square centimetres. The microscopic villi increase this figure by approximately 600 times to make the total area for absorption 45 million square centimetres or 4,500 metres, a huge figure. The term 'small intestine' can be confusing for it is over 20 feet long and has the area of three tennis courts placed next to each other. We have plenty of room, therefore, to absorb the nutrients from food but we must be sure that the nutrients of the food are accessible to the process of absorption. This means that we must chew our food thoroughly to break it down properly and relax during our meals so that the food has the correct concentration of acids, enzymes, and hormones to ensure proper digestion.

The large intestine contains myriads of bacteria, most of which are harmless and in fact necessary to provide certain B group vitamins which we cannot live without. Strong laxatives and antibiotics sweep these bacteria out, thus depriving the body of important products. We should use them only when it is absolutely necessary.

Key to health

A great many disorders are connected directly or indirectly with the malfunction of the digestive system. It is said that disorders of the digestive system are the root cause of many of our modern day diseases such as heart disease, cancer, arthritis, etc. Some authorities go so far as to claim that poor digestion and a bad stomach are the root cause of all our problems. Of course, behind poor digestion is an inability of the mind to digest the situations of life and to metabolize the problems correctly. You must have noticed for yourself that when you are experiencing digestive troubles you tend to be pessimistic and easily irritated. Conversely, a healthy digestive system allows one to be cheerful, happy and optimistic.

Yoga is the key to a relaxed, efficient, harmonious digestive system. It is the way by which the body systems can be tuned to a state of good health. With yoga as a guide we come to a complete understanding of what proper digestion can mean to our whole way of life. A strong digestive system means energy and vitality, it reflects a positive lifestyle.

3

Ayurvedic Physiology

Ayurveda, the ancient healing science of India, was devised thousands of years ago by sages and seers as a means to help suffering humanity. At this time there was no sophisticated technological equipment, so that medical experts had to rely on the skilful manipulation of their own inner equipment: intuition, analytical reasoning, intelligence and keen perception combined with observation of external disease manifestations. This fusion of the subjective with the objective is the meditative process. Out of this grew a system of great complexity and a great ability to cure disease.

The doshas

Ayurveda regards food as the life of all living creatures because it nourishes the components of the body. Ayurveda classifies life according to principles called doshas. There are three main doshas:

1. Kapha, translated as phlegm or mucus, but referring more to protoplasm, is the water which forms the ground structure of the body tissues. This fluid sometimes referred to as *soma,* the water of life, is said to bind the limbs and organs, and provide the connecting, nourishing, developing and fortifying functions. It maintains the well-being of the body by its lubricating action. Its properties are cold, viscous and heavy. It is the principle of potential energy storage and is also associated with the power of perseverance.

2. Pitta is translated as bile or gall and is closely related with temperament. It is the fire that exists in the body, acting on matter to transform it. This results in digestion, power of perception, body temperature, healthy appearance, emotions (fear, anger, joy), clarity, and also their opposite when pitta is not functioning properly. Its properties are heat and transformation.

3. Vata is translated as wind, implying movement. It is related to mental energy. In the body it is divided into the five pranas (i) *udana* – located in the extremities: arms, legs and head, (ii) *prana* – from the throat to the heart, (iii) *samana* – from the heart to the navel, (iv) *apana* – from the navel to the perineum, (v) *vyana* – pervades the whole body. Vata initiates upward and downward movements. It is the guiding force for consciousness and the sensation of the sense organs. As well as organizing the elements of the body, it is the storage battery for speech, the principle of synthesis, the cause of feeling and perception and the source of excitement and stimulation. Vata fans the gastric fire and purifies the channels of the body.

In order to maintain health and a good digestive system, the doshas must be properly balanced. The proportion and ratio of the various doshas change with each season and also at different times of the day. Food must therefore be taken seasonally and in the correct amount and proportion for each dosha. This ensures that deficiencies and excesses are corrected, otherwise the doshas become unbalanced.

Digestive fire

The digestive fire is essential for good health. When it becomes weak, indigestion and other disorders set in because of poor nourishment. Proper digestion requires that the various 'fires' of the body – the chemicals, acids, enzymes and other digestive juices are in their correct proportion to maintain growth, strength, complexion, happiness and to prolong the existence of a healthy body.

18

The process of digestion occurs because of heat from various chemical reactions, water which softens the digesting food and air which fans the fire. Fire is the most important element out of which fine substances imbued with energy are produced. In medical terms this fine essence of food is composed of the amino acids, small sugars, etc. which are necessary for the life systems.

Digestion follows a basic process. The ayurvedic and yogic terms used here must be seen in their correct relationship to the digestive system:

1. The life breath, prana, seizes the food and sends it down to the stomach in the swallowing act.
2. The digestive fire stirred up by samana, burns and blazes forth in the stomach when nutritious food is taken. At the same time the solid food is dissolved by liquid gastric juices and softened by oily matter (mucus). The digestive fire is said to be below and to cook the gastric content like rice in a pot, converting it into essence *(rasa)* and wastes *(mal)*. A foamy reaction is produced by kapha (mucus) and after this the half-digested food becomes sour (acids).
3. It then passes out of the stomach and reacts with pitta (bile) from the liver.
4. In the intestines the food is eventually dried by fire into a compact mass. During the process, vata (wind, prana) is produced by a bitter and astringent reaction.
5. The digested food travels by arteries to nourish the tissues.
6. The wastes of the body form in the digestive and metabolic processes. Faeces and urine come from food and water. Mucus is produced from food and water. Mucus is produced from the essence (rasa) derived from digestion of food and is expelled in sneezing, etc. Bile (pitta) is derived from blood and expelled with faeces. The wastes from the metabolism of flesh come out in the ears as wax, the eyes as tears, the nostrils as phlegm. Fat waste comes out in sweat. Hair and nails come from bone. Oiliness in the skin comes from the marrow. These 'wastes' have their own specific function and thereby sustain the body

19

as long as they are not produced in excess. When excessive they pollute, weaken and cause disease.

Ayurvedic physiology goes on to state that each element of the food has its own specific elemental fire which can be interpreted to mean its own chemical reaction. Thus each element gives a still finer essence which is used to form another body tissue in the following increasingly more subtle order: essence is taken into the blood to produce flesh which then produces fat, bone, marrow, semen and finally energy (*ojas*). Each element also gives off a waste. The elements also retain their own substance which is driven by the pranas to their own specific destination.

Feeding the fire

Food is fuel for the digestive fire and therefore must be pure, well combined and in correct quantity. The amount of food one needs to eat depends on one's digestive power. We must discover our own capacity and set ourselves a standard amount to eat at each meal. Few people, however, can stop eating at the point of satisfaction or a little short of it. Constantly eating beyond this point vitiates the digestive fire. Undigested food is worse than no food and becomes a detriment to our health. The body is the product of the food taken in and all materials used as food are compounded from the five elements:

1. Earth – used for building bones, nails, teeth, muscle and skin.
2. Water – supplies substances for fat, blood, lymph, urine and sweat. These substances are inactive, soft, viscous and slimy.
3. Fire – makes the body radiant.
4. Air – maintains exhalation and inhalation, eyelid movements, contraction and expansion, excitement and incitement, and movement.
5. Ether – supplies the pores and channels of the body.
   Food is also divided into ten dual qualities: (i) heavy-light, (ii) cold-hot, (iii) oily-dry, (iv) mild-sharp, (v) compact-expansive,

(vi) soft-hard, (vii) cleansing-slimy, (viii) smooth-rough, (ix) minute-gross, (x) solid-liquid.

Light and heavy are the most important qualities of food. Light food contains the elements of wind and heat and therefore is the best to maintain the digestive fire. It is less injurious when taken to satiety. Bitter tasting food is lightest, followed by pungent and sour tasting food. Heavy food contains the elements of earth and water and therefore dampens the digestive fire. It is injurious when taken in excess. Sweet tasting foods are the heaviest type. Of course, a well balanced diet is essential and contains a mix of different types of light and heavy foods.

Heating and cooling foods are also important in terms of maintaining digestion. Heat producing foods are saline, sour and pungent, while cooling foods are sweet, bitter and astringent. Oily foods contain the element of earth and water and are lubricating and cooling. Drying foods contain air; softening foods, water and ether; cleansing foods, air and earth. By understanding the qualities of foods we are eating, we can manipulate and adjust the body's functions in the same way as we would the control on a gas stove.

Practical ayurveda

Ayurveda proposes a system of synthesizing food and digestion so that a balanced nourishing diet can be incorporated into our lifestyle. To ensure that your intake will balance the doshas choose natural foods in season. To maintain the digestive fire, eat light meals and never overload. These simple rules are the basis for healthy living.

Two meals per day, one between 9 a.m. and 12 p.m. and the other between 5 p.m. and 7 p.m. are recommended. The appetite is stimulated just before meals with a little salt or ginger. Other suggestions are given regarding diet and how to sit at meals. Sitting cross-legged on the floor is said to enhance the energies in the abdomen by bringing them up from the legs. Moderation in drinking is also important – drinking before meals gives one a tendency towards thinness and after meals towards stoutness. Further recommendations include careful hygiene of the mouth and a short walk after meals. By following these suggestions, digestion is improved.

The recommended diet includes: various cereals (especially rice and wheat), fruit, vegetables, nuts, ginger, garlic, salt, pure water (rainwater is said to be the best), milk, oil, butter, honey and sugar cane. The amount of each depends on individual capacity. A balanced (sattwic) approach to diet helps us to balance our whole lives. It can actually be a means of enhancing consciousness if approached correctly. A simple, pure diet keeps our digestive system healthy and this has a positive, beneficial effect on our mental state, personality and interpersonal relationships. At the same time it is only possible to live a simple life if our minds are pure and relaxed, and this cannot be achieved by diet alone, but by a combination of yogic practices and dietary discrimination.

4

Food for Thought

Few people realize just how important food is in their lives. It is not until we deliberately try to stop eating that we see how many hours are spent daily in buying, preparing and washing up after the thrice-daily ritual of eating.

The subject of diet and nutrition has become increasingly popular. Thousands of books and magazines are dedicated to this subject. Though they mean well, many of these publications tend to make people worry excessively about their food habits and whether they are consuming the right foods in sufficient quantity to avoid vitamin deficiency. Food neurosis is actually far worse than failing to get enough nutrients. Therefore, we emphasize: 'try to avoid food fads and fanaticism', and the best way to do this is to learn about nutrients and the body. Then you will realize that all the nutrients which the body needs are to be found in a wide range of food types. If you eat a varied diet, you will get all your necessary food requirements. Occasionally during times of stress you may need to supplement your intake; however, a balanced diet and yoga will give you everything you need.

NUTRIENTS AND THE BODY

By learning the basic facts about diet and the constituents of different foods, we are better able to decide what we want and need to eat. Taste, desire and fantasy then play a lesser role to objectivity, knowledge and understanding. In this way food becomes part of a scientific approach to life, rather than just a means of satisfying hunger. This is the yogic approach to nutrition.

There are five main components of food: carbohydrates, fats, proteins, vitamins and minerals.

Carbohydrates and fats

These provide our body with energy, about 75% of which is converted into heat and maintains the body temperature. We need fewer carbohydrates and fats in hot weather, but in winter our digestive fire burns like a volcano and we need to eat more. The rest of the energy is used by the muscles, motor system, heart, brain and internal organs. Fats also form a protective layer, shielding organs from injury and allowing a storage of energy for future use. Overconsumption of these foods, however, leads to overweight. Butter and oils are almost pure fat, while sugar is 100% carbohydrate. Potato, rice, bread and grains contain mostly carbohydrate along with vitamins and minerals, and very little fat.

Proteins

Out of these remarkable materials the body tissues are built. Proteins repair worn out tissues and this process goes on continually. They are also necessary for the production of essential special substances called immunoglobulins that help build up the body's resistance to disease. Protein is found in meat, milk, cheese, fish, eggs, grains, legumes, nuts, etc.

Mineral salts

These essential elements are present in certain foods in minute quantities. Phosphorus and calcium are required in relatively large amounts for building bones and teeth, and activating muscles and the brain. Iron helps the blood to carry oxygen through the body and it is used by the blood cells. It is found in eggs, raisins, spinach, wholegrains, apricots, potatoes, meat and liver. Iodine is used by the

24

thyroid gland to control the whole process of metabolism. It is found in iodized salt, seafood and vegetables. Salt, in the form of sodium chloride, is essential for the maintenance of normal acid to base balance. Too much salt in the body raises the blood pressure and causes swelling in the legs so only a moderate amount in the diet is recommended.

Vitamins

Vitamins are engaged in many different and diversified functions. Vitamin A is used in all the organs of the body, especially the respiratory, digestive and urinary tracts. It keeps the mucus membrane of the nose, throat and windpipe strong and healthy, in this way helping to prevent colds and other infections. Vitamin A keeps the skin smooth and clear and is perhaps best known for its use in the maintenance of vision, a lack of which can cause night blindness. The best sources are carrots, fruits, vegetables, cream, butter, wholemilk and egg yolk.

The vitamin B complex has more than a dozen different components. B_1 or thiamine is important and is concerned with nerves and muscles. It is thought that a lack of thiamine causes alcoholics to suffer from nervous system and liver degeneration. Without thiamine the body would be in a constant state of aches and pains, swelling, and heart and liver failure. Thiamine is most prevalent in liver, brewers yeast, peanuts, wholegrains, meat, and eggs. Riboflavin, another important member, is necessary for skin, eyes and digestion. Niacin is also important for digestion. All the elements necessary for this essential component are found in wholegrain, milk, cheese, eggs and liver.

Vitamin C is the great healing vitamin essential for the building of connective tissues, bones, small blood vessels, teeth and gums. A lack of this vitamin causes scurvy. It is found in fresh fruits (especially guava and citrus), green leafy vegetables, potatoes and tomatoes. Vitamin C is destroyed by cooking so we must assume that any cooked food does not contain much of it.

Vitamin D is necessary for the development of strong, healthy bones. A deficiency causes rickets (softening of the bones), but this is rare as the body can manufacture its own supply from sunshine and fresh air interacting with oils in the skin. It can also be found in milk, eggs and vegetable oils.

Vitamin E helps the nucleus of the cells and the reproductive function. It is extremely valuable in all heart and artery diseases as it reduces the need of the tissue cells for oxygen, prevents clotting (thrombosis) and dilates the smallest blood vessels. It aids the healing of burns and ulcers, prevents formation of hard scar tissues and softens old scars. Muscles, including those of the heart, are strengthened by vitamin E, blood circulation is improved and production of the sexual hormones is regulated. It is found in wholegrains, green leafy vegetables, soya beans, tomatoes and eggs.

Vitamins are found in a great variety of foods, so there is really no need to take extra vitamin supplements if you are eating well. At times of stress more vitamin B and C may be required and a supplement may be useful.

DIETARY SUGGESTIONS

Most people who have any degree of sensitivity know which diet is best for them. The body tells us in so many different ways. For example, if the breath smells bad, then the food is not digesting properly and is acting like a poison. Our appetite also tells us what we need to eat and when we start eating, the taste buds of the tongue tell us whether the food is good for us or not. The trouble is that too often we just don't listen!

Better alternatives
The following chart will enable you to avoid foods that are either detrimental to digestion or are processed in such a way as to lose their prana and nutritional value. The alternatives given are far better for the health.

26

Food to avoid: Denatured foods: white flour, white bread, cakes and buns, polished white rice. White sugar, sweets, jam, sweet syrups, fruit in syrups, light treacle, heavily sugared drinks and glucose drinks. Fats and oils of animal origin, saturated acid fats. Heat treated, canned foods, processed foods in which artificial sweeteners, flavourings and chemical preservatives are used (always read the small type on labels before purchasing).

Food to use: Whole wheat, barley, rye or cornflour bread, whole or partially polished rice. Honey, brown sugar, molasses, black treacle, fresh fruit. Vegetable oils and clarified butter Fresh foods, naturally processed foods like dried fruit or lentils and organically grown products.

Health hints

Here are a few basic suggestions which can help you and your family on the road to good health:
1. Buy fresh foods and store at a cool temperature. Fruits and vegetables in season are cheap and also best suited to the needs of the body.
2. Rinse all the dirt and chemical sprays off the surface of fruits and vegetables. There is no need to scrub away the skin or peel the skins as they have a great deal of nutrients and also add roughage to the diet.
3. Steaming or baking is better than frying or boiling. In the ashram vegetables are fried first in a little vegetable oil, then some water is added and they are steamed until soft. This gives them a good flavour and makes them easy to digest.
4. If you eat meat, do not fry it. Remove all fat before cooking in order to reduce the amount of saturated fatty acids; this is better for the heart and blood vessels. Boil, bake or broil meat.
5. Avoid large amounts of fat, oil or ghee.
6. Use salt sparingly, more in summer and less in winter. Try to season your food with herbs, lemon juice or natural soya sauce.

7. Do not overcook

8. Prepare food just before serving in order to maintain the maximum prana and nutrition.

9. Cook with care in order to increase prana. Make meals attractive and tasty to stimulate the appetite and digestive enzymes.

10. Keep meals simple. Remember, all the different foods you put on your plate will mix in your stomach.

11. Take meals at regular intervals.

12. Do not eat in between meals.

13. Bathe before meals or not until half an hour after meals, as bathing diverts the blood from the stomach and intestines to the skin.

14. When eating always take small mouthfuls. Chew each mouthful carefully and chew fried foods a little longer.

15. Eliminate problems from your mind during the meal. Do not eat food when you are tense or angry. Calmness is conducive to good digestion.

16. Take food with the attitude that it is health-giving, the gift of God or nature.

17. Only take as much as you need; never overburden the digestive system.

The body needs a little food and little fasting if it is to grow in a balanced way, just as a plant will die if it is watered too much, and does not get enough sun.

5

All in Good Taste

No organ causes so much trouble as the tongue. It can get us into endless strife outside as well as inside. Talking and eating rank amongst the hardest body processes to control. Indeed it is the tongue which is responsible for many of the quarrels and misunderstandings in the world, as well as for much of the dietary indiscretion which leads to indigestion and further ill health. The tongue is a channel by which the mind communicates with the outside world, satisfying inner needs and desires as well as expressing thoughts and feelings. The tongue is so powerful an organ that some people eat only to satisfy it, without even thinking of the other 32 feet of digestive tract.

Protected by the teeth, the tongue is potentially a doorway to higher, blissful experience. With control it can produce gentle speech and beautiful song. It can savour tasty dishes, or in a yogic sadhana can taste the nectar of immortality *(amrit)*. Directed outward towards the world, or upward and inward as in khechari mudra, the tongue can be a useful and amazingly intricate tool for exploring both the outer and inner worlds. The tongue is also a sensitive mirror of body health. A perfectly healthy body will have a rosy pink tongue with no coating. Any digestive upset, no matter how mild, will produce a fine white fur on top of the tongue. In more obvious disease the coating becomes thicker and darker, as in fevers. The tongue should be cleaned every morning while cleaning the teeth, as this prevents accumulated toxins from going back into the body.

Taste receptors

The sense of taste is mediated by taste receptors situated on the upper portion of the tongue and also to a lesser extent on the palate, pharynx and tonsils. Medically speaking, the receptors are said to send four different kinds of taste sensations to the brain and mind, though the exact mechanisms are not known. The taste sensations are scattered mainly over the surface of the tongue. The tip of the tongue is sensitive to all four modalities: sweet, bitter, sour, salty – but mainly to sweet. The sides of the tongue are sensitive mainly to sour (acid) things but also to salt. The back of the tongue is sensitive to bitter.

The taste we experience is a result of the combination of these primary tastes and various smells, as all foods have different quantities and qualities of the basic types. Sensations of heat, cold, touch and pain are also sent from the tongue to the brain, and these play an important role in the evaluation of taste.

Ayurvedic analysis

Ayurveda describes six different tastes, adding pungent and astringent to the medical four. It states the nutritive power of food depends to a large extent on taste. The ayurvedic classification of taste is:

1. *Sweet* increases energy in the body and stimulates the senses. It produces moisture, cold and heaviness, and can therefore be said to increase tamo guna. It is composed of the earth and water elements.
2. *Saline* helps digestion, removes excess wind (vata), secretes phlegm (kapha) and is moist and warm. It is composed of the water and fire elements.
3. *Bitter* is unpalatable to the mind but it sharpens the appetite, assists the digestion and helps eliminate toxins. Foods with this quality are karella, wormwood, quinine

30

and hops. It is dry, cool and light, being composed of the air and ether elements, and increases sattwa guna.

4. *Sour* is the acidic, tart taste found in vinegar, lemons, the juice of unripe fruit (sour apples, sour grapes) and products of fermentation (unsweetened yoghurt or curd).
5. *Pungent* is more a quality of taste than a taste itself and is said to be the product of irritation. It is a sharp, hot, pricking, biting quality as found in chilli, radish, ginger and other spices. Having the elements of fire and air, it is said to increase the digestive fire and rajo guna.
6. *Astringent* qualities restore harmony by contracting the soft organic textures and binding the body elements together. Lemon peel has this effect, making the mouth feel dry and contracted; it is also found in unripe fruit. Having the elements of earth and fire, it is dry, cool and heavy.

From this classification of taste we can see that certain foods will have specific effects on the body. We can affect our temperament, body-type and so on just by the food we eat. For example excessive amounts of sweet food, when not balanced with the other aspects of taste, increase the heaviness of the body and make the senses function more strongly. Thus the material nature begins to predominate and to affect the mind, making it heavy and tamasic. Of course, the desire for sweet food reflects a certain state of consciousness, but by indulging in our desires we only increase the tendency. A desire for chillies, on the other hand, reflects a different state of consciousness. Chillies and other hot food tend to make the body more rajasic and energetic. Bitter foods balance the diet and increase sattwa by purifying the body. Bitterness takes the mind away from the senses so that it is able to objectify them.

A sattwic or pure diet is a balanced, bland diet. However, we can use chillies and sweet food if desired, and maintain sattwa as long as we are not excessive in any direction. When we practise yoga, diet is an adjunct to the raising of consciousness, but this does not mean that strict limitations must be imposed. Control over the senses is a spontaneous outcome of regular yoga practice.

31

Taste and nutrition

Taste is not just for pleasure, enabling us to enjoy a wider range of sensual experiences, but also has a protective value. Experiments by Richter show that taste plays a critical role in nutrition and in maintaining a constant internal environment.[1] Rats suffering from a shortage of some nutrient, due to endocrine abnormalities, craved and selectively ate those foods which replaced their deficiency. Taste provided the sensory cue by which these discriminative selections were made. Animals whose taste nerves are cut are no longer able to correct deficiencies by regulating diet.

The sense of taste is therefore a means of tuning into our deeper instinctive and intuitive side. It can point out what we need and what we want, but it is up to our own inner sense of discrimination to decide what is the correct way to proceed. If we are aware or sensitive enough the taste receptors will signal 'bad' food or harmful food and we can spit it out before it enters the body. Of course, what we experience depends to a large extent on our previous mental conditioning. For example, if we have had a bad experience from eating pumpkin, we may tend to remember this every time we eat pumpkin, which then becomes a 'bad' food. These experiences clutter our perception and make it difficult to discriminate between truly harmful food and imaginary danger or individual dislike. A system is required to find our way out of the morass of past experiences and conditioning so that we can sense and feel clearly without an intervening screen from the past.

Yoga provides techniques which increase sensitivity and mental clarity. These methods uncork the bottle of the past and release the hold which past experiences have on us; they are then able to bubble out by themselves leaving us free from their impressions.

Some authorities maintain that pleasant tasting food is essential for life and is the first prerequisite for good digestion because of its effects on the mind. For the gastric and intestinal secretions to flow, complex interactions of the brain and nervous system are required and this determines the quality of digestion. Eating tasteless, monotonous food becomes a stress rather than a pleasure. Tasty, pleasant, nourishing food stimulates and encourages a plentiful outpouring of the digestive juices. Therefore, the nutritive properties of food depend not only on the quality of the food itself, but also upon the way in which it is prepared and the atmosphere in which it is eaten. One's mental attitude is also of great importance for good digestion.

The psychology of taste

We realize the importance of taste when we look into the psychology of the idiom 'in good taste'. We judge the world around us by how it tastes to us. For example:

1. *Sweetness* is associated with those things that are pleasing and agreeable – sweet words. We may enjoy the sweetness. A sweet person is gracious, sympathetic, amiable and understanding. One may by sweet-spoken, sweet-souled. The term 'to be sweet on someone' means that you are strongly attracted to that person. You may then do some sweet-talking and that person may become your sweet-heart.

2. *Sour* is the opposite of sweet. Sour people are cross, crabby, morose, unpleasant. One who wears a 'sour coun-tenance' is likely to be jealous, unsympathetic and irritable.

3. *Bitterness* is said to be a disagreeable taste and some people associate it with medicine. A bitter experience is painful and distressing to the body, mind and soul, but from it we learn some of the most valuable lessons in life. We speak of bitter grief, bitter feelings, bitter tears, bitter scorn, the bitter side of life. Keats wrote "Ah, bitter chill it was!" emphasizing the coldness associated with it.

4. *Salt* implies earthiness and a practical nature. In food, salt is added for flavour and seasoning, and a salty nature is full of the wit and piquancy which seasons life. To be 'worth one's salt' means to be efficient and deserving.

Enjoying with awareness

The sense of taste permeates life at many levels. As an exercise in awareness, pick out the different tastes of your next meal and enjoy, savour and watch them fully. That is the tantric approach to conquering the sense of taste and bringing it fully under our control. Instead of trying to cut off the senses forcibly as is enjoined by some spiritual aspirants, tantra tells us to enjoy all those things we like and not to suppress. By maintaining awareness while we are stimulating our senses, we trace their origin back to the mind. In this way, detachment develops and we learn to control our senses, turning them on and off at will. Awareness also provides the solvent for desires, ambitions and frustrations that too often manoeuvre and lead us to misuse our taste buds.

Taste, according to yogic psychophysiology, is associated with swadhisthana chakra, the centre of pleasure gratification and preservation of the species. Pleasure gratification, which is a strong motivating force in all of us, can manifest in two main ways – through food and through sex. If either of these aspects is overactive because of an imbalance in hormonal secretions, excessive stimulation of the nervous system or strong subconscious desire, then it may overpower our will and result in overindulgence. We cannot stop doing what we desire to do, for there is no conscious willpower to say 'No'. We can, however, practise yogic techniques which balance the swadhisthana chakra system and thereby regulate excessive desire. Meditation allows us to become aware of the role of craving for tastes and other associated pleasures in our lives. In this way we gain knowledge about ourselves, which is the first step in developing control.

Taste sadhana

The tongue is used in many yogic practices to help control the fluctuations of the mind. The technique of khechari mudra, folding the tongue backwards, is used to stimulate the brain and to signal the mind that we wish to turn our attention inwards, creating a psychic gesture. Khechari is a tantric technique allowing us to transcend the senses and the mind through the sense of taste itself. We use the tongue, which is usually pointed outwards towards the external world, as a means to travel in and up to the spiritual heights.

In the full form of khechari mudra, the tongue is folded back into the pharynx and then reaches upwards to touch a gland at the back of the nose, just below the eyebrow centre, which secretes either a poison or a nectar, depending on our state of consciousness. By practising khechari mudra we can actually taste this secretion.

Most people practise nabho mudra, the simplified version of khechari mudra, in which the tongue is held against the soft palate. Over a period of time it becomes more and more supple so that it can slowly approximate the advanced form.

In the ancient yogic scriptures it is stated that:

When the yogi now curls his tongue upward and back, he is able to close the place where the three paths meet. The bending back of the tongue is khechari mudra and the closing of three paths is akasha chakra. The yogi who remains but half a minute in this position is free from illness, old age and death. He who has mastered khechari mudra is not afflicted with disease, death, sloth, hunger, thirst and swooning.

Hatha Yoga Pradipika 8: 36–39

The body becomes beautiful, samadhi is attained, and the tongue touching the holes in the roof of the mouth obtains various juices first he experiences a salty taste, then alkaline, then bitter, then astringent, then he feels the taste of butter, then ghee, then milk, then curd, then whey, then honey, then palm juice and lastly arises the taste of nectar.

Gherand Samhita 3: 30–32

According to these texts, the sense of taste can be used in the practice of khechari mudra as an instrument to measure the state of our physical and mental purity, thereby aiding us on the path to spiritual attainment.

In heightened states of consciousness definite changes occur in the brain, endocrinal and chemical structure of the body. The glands mirror this change, so that when khechari is performed we taste the sweetness that is within us. This state is actually monitored in the brain and the experience is said to be so overwhelming that one drop of this nectar confers bliss and immortality.

6

Vegetarianism and Yoga

It is my view that the vegetarian manner of living, by its purely physical effect on the human temperament, would most beneficially influence the lot of mankind.

Albert Einstein

The most controversial issue regarding diet is whether or not to be vegetarian. The generally understood and accepted definition of vegetarianism is abstention from animal flesh and related products. However, various forms of vegetarianism have arisen because of conflicting opinions regarding the suitability of eating milk, eggs, fish and dairy products. Strict vegetarians, or vegans, do not eat eggs or fish, while many people who consider themselves to be practising vegetarians do. Thus the definition of vegetarianism depends on individual interpretation.

There are many arguments for and against vegetarianism. Most people go to one extreme or the other and the subject is generally discussed dogmatically and with too much emphasis on the moral aspects. Therefore, in order to gain a balanced perspective, we must examine the question from both viewpoints. Here are some of the arguments in favour of meat.

Meat is an excellent source of first class protein containing all the essential amino acids for proper growth and maintenance of the body. Amino acids are the building blocks for all body proteins. Vegetable is a second class protein because it does not contain all the essential amino acids. However, if we mix grains and legumes in the ration of four parts grain to one part legumes, all the amino acids are available. For example, rice and dal or baked beans on wholemeal toast in the correct ratio supply the body with all it needs in the way of protein.

Meat is high in vitamin B_{12} while a vegetarian diet is considered to be low. However, it has been shown that there is sufficient B_{12} in green vegetables to supply the needs of the body. Vitamin B_{12} is also found in yeast, yeast extract, eggs, milk, yoghurt and fermented food such as bean curd or pakhal (fermented rice). Some vegetarians claim that because certain bacteria produce B_{12}, it is possible to achieve a state in which friendly bacteria can be induced to live in the intestines producing our own B_{12}, as occurs in certain ruminant animals. These people state that a meat diet is detrimental to the vitamin B_{12} production in the body.

Among the arguments against meat, one of the most thought-provoking is the fact that many modern methods of slaughter result in meat that is contaminated by various chemicals such as the hormone adrenaline. Animals are highly stressed at the time of slaughter and large amounts of adrenaline are released into the bloodstream. This chemical remains in the blood and meat and is ingested into our system, charging us with stress and creating a nervous, aggressive, fearful state.

The use of artificial methods to stimulate an animal's growth is common throughout the world. Antibiotics, hormones, vaccines and other substances are given to animals by mouth or injection. These also remain in the meat and when consumed they unbalance the neuroendocrine system.

The flesh of dead animals can be a breeding ground for many different types of bacteria. It is known that bad meat and flesh produce some of the most powerful poisons known. Meat must be cooked properly, especially when there is inadequate refrigeration. Apart from the poisons introduced by man, all of the animal's natural waste products are found in the cells of its tissues. Expelling these toxins and waste products consumed in meat products imposes an extra burden on our organs of elimination.

Surveys in various countries have shown that those with high levels of meat consumption, particularly New Zealand, USA, Australia and other industrially developed countries, have the highest rate of colon cancer. In countries that did not consume much meat, such as Nigeria, the level of colon cancer was negligible. Demographical studies are difficult to interpret, so these results are not conclusive, but they suggest that excessive meat plays a role in causing cancer. Many other conditions have been associated with meat intake, for example arteriosclerosis, rheumatism, haemorrhoids and constipation.

The body requires a certain amount of protein to build up and rejuvenate all the worn out cells. If more than this amount is ingested, the excess is utilized for providing energy needs. This is not very economical in terms of energy expenditure however, as the total amount of energy spent on turning protein into energy is more than the amount of energy gained from the extra protein. Thus we lose energy in the process, which is why protein diets are good for losing weight. The proteins that are converted in this manner tend to leave behind certain residues or 'ashes' in the body as by-products. These have to be eliminated by the kidneys, lungs and skin, thus placing a greater load on these organs. This is also the reason why people who eat meat have a strong body odour and when they change over to a vegetarian diet this odour leaves them.

Throughout the ages, sages and philosophers have advocated vegetarianism as the preferred way of life. Archimedes and many other Greek philosophers urged people to become vegetarian. George Bernard Shaw told people that if they wanted to eat meat they should first be able to watch their food being slaughtered and made ready for the dinner table.

They recommended vegetarianism because they knew about the intimate relationship between the body and mind, and that what we eat has a definite effect on our state of mind. Vegetarianism has been shown to promote inner calmness and harmony between the body and the mind, while eating meat has been linked with internal tension, disharmony and arousal of passion. This does not mean that vegetarianism will immediately give you a peaceful mind, but it will definitely aid the process while yogic techniques perform the main work.

Vegetarianism and digestive problems

Vegetarianism is the basis of a sattwic diet which increases vitality as it is light and easy to digest. Meat, on the other hand, is heavy, rajasic and takes a lot of energy to digest. From the point of view of digestive problems a vegetarian diet goes a long way in aiding therapeutic techniques. In some cases diet alone is therapeutic and the yogic exercises only act to speed up the natural healing processes. Constipation, for example, is due in many cases to a low residue meat diet, which does not have the necessary bulk to stimulate movement of the intestines. As a result, haemorrhoids and perhaps even cancer can also form.

If you do not have any digestive problems and you are eating meat, then perhaps this is the correct diet for your occupation and lifestyle. However, a meat-eater with indigestion will greatly benefit from at least a short-term vegetarian diet. Of course many vegetarians also get indigestion, but from our experience it is much easier to cure these people with minor dietary changes than it is to cure those who eat meat. This seems to be because vegetarians are used to lighter, more easily digestible food and thus have more reserve energy in their system. Vegetarianism combined with regular and sensible eating habits and the appropriate yoga practices will definitely relieve digestive problems. Try to adopt a vegetarian diet while you are using the techniques given here, even if it is only for three months.

During this time you may find the benefits of vegetarianism outweigh the disadvantages.

As a staple diet vegetarianism does not have to be strict and rigid. Eating meat occasionally on social occasions or with friends does no harm in the long term. Manu, the codifier of laws in ancient India, summed up the sensible approach to the whole subject as follows: "There is no wrong in eating meat or drinking wine, but abstention gives many benefits."

The how of vegetarianism

When making the changeover to a vegetarian diet, it is important to know what else to use in order to maintain the body's protein supply, as well as other aspects of diet. Soya beans are known to be richer in protein than meat, weight for weight. This is often a surprise to many people. Soya beans have been used by the Chinese and other oriental people for centuries. Nearly 40% of the soya bean is pure protein. This is about twice that of meat and four times that of eggs, wheat and other cereals. There are many other fine foods that contain a high percentage of protein, the most widely known being nuts of all types, lentils, sunflower seeds, milk, yoghurt, cheese, as well as all other dairy products.

One thing is certain, you will always obtain your protein and all other nutrients if you eat a reasonably varied vegetarian diet. People often say that vegetarian food is tasteless and monotonous compared to non-vegetarian food. This is only true when there is lack of imagination and unskilful preparation on the part of the cook. There are various vegetarian cookbooks available which give a wide variety of meals that are every bit as tasty as non-vegetarian cooking.

YOGIC VIEW

It is assumed that vegetarianism is an integral part of yogic practice. This is only partially true however, for while yoga views vegetarianism as the most beneficial system of

41

nutrition, it does not for an instant insist that practitioners of yoga become vegetarians. Although becoming vegetarian is preparation for higher forms of yoga, non-vegetarians are heartily accepted as practitioners of yoga. Yoga advises but does not preach vegetarianism.

Yogic practices in themselves have nothing whatsoever to do with diet, whether vegetarian or non-vegetarian. The aim of yoga is to expand the awareness and awaken the prana shakti which can sustain the body even in the absence of a so-called nutritious diet. By practising yoga, both mental and physical health are improved, regardless of whether one is vegetarian or non-vegetarian. At the same time yoga recognizes that food is as much a necessity for the aspirant as mental, emotional and spiritual nourishment. In yoga a simple diet is used to fuel the physical body (*annamaya kosha*), and hatha yoga to remove its impurities. Pranayama charges the vital energy body (*pranamaya kosha*) while meditation develops the mental and psychic bodies (*manomaya and vijnanamaya koshas*). As far as making food a path to higher consciousness however, no diet on its own has yet succeeded, and the yogic diet is no exception.

Many people are surprised to find that there is no fixed yogic diet; it varies from climate to climate, season to season and sadhana to sadhana. Perhaps the ideal yogic diet can be summed up as the most natural and simplest to purchase, to prepare and digest.

Sattwic diet
That diet which augments the balanced state of the body and mind is said to be sattwic. In India this diet consists of fruits, nuts, milk (and milk products), steamed vegetables, cooked grains, beans and lentils. These foods are said to increase sattwa in the body because they are light, simple and supply all the correct nutrients. At the same time they increase our mental and physical vitality so that we can more easily experience peace, bliss, lightness and clarity of mind.

Perhaps the best sattwic preparation for yogis is khichari, which is common in India but can also be easily prepared in most countries around the world. It is made of rice or wheat, lentils and vegetables all cooked together into a light, easily digested meal which provides all nutrients (except vitamin C) and gives us plenty of energy.

Rajasic food differs from sattwic food in that it is prepared with many spices and plenty of ghee or oil. This food is heavier and creates restlessness in the mind. Meat and fish are rajasic. Some yogis also say that milk is rajasic because it excites the sexual hormones and makes one stronger physically but not mentally.

Tamasic foods are old and stale, lowering the energy and producing inertia. Foods which are not cooked or chewed well also fall into this category as do dead or highly processed foods.

By avoiding rajasic and tamasic foods as far as possible and sticking mainly to a sattwic diet, we can gradually alter the inner body chemistry. All the digestive enzymes and nutritional properties are renewed when the foods consumed are light and full of energy.

Discipline

Why are so many people sick today? Why are so few in control of their bodies, minds and lives? Probably the main cause is a lack of willpower, discipline and common sense. Many people let their tongues rule their lives. When discipline is cultivated through yoga and the bodily systems become more balanced, we begin to naturally and spontaneously like those things that are good for us and reject those that upset our bodies and minds. The desire for sattwa develops from discipline.

When we control the mind we control the physical body. Vitality is conserved and concentrated. The nervous system is calmed and the hormones of the pituitary are stored and then used more effectively and appropriately. These energy reserves are available for sensual activity but can also be transformed into spiritual energy, prana shakti or ojas. As we begin to concentrate our mind and become more sattwic, the body processes become balanced and fewer precious nutrients are wasted. When, through samadhi, we transcend sattwa altogether, the actual energy source changes and the body no longer requires food.

Diet and metabolism

We are constantly taking food in and expelling wastes as part of the metabolic process. The sattwic diet maintains an even metabolism – input equals output; absorption of nutrients equals elimination of wastes. No excess or heavy demands are made on the body and thus health is maintained.

A rajasic diet increases metabolism and activates the nervous and endocrine systems. It demands a lot of attention as one must constantly satisfy the desires and cravings that arise from this overactivity. A tamasic diet, on the other hand, makes one underactive, lazy and dull. Parts of the physical organism may actually shut down due to it. Both rajasic and tamasic diets lead to disease. When they are replaced by a sattwic diet the metabolism and the whole body function are rebalanced.

Changing with the seasons

The ancient yogic scriptures have given us extensive advice on how to maintain a sattwic diet. The recommendation vary with climate, season and personality type.

- *Climate*: Whatever foods nature provides will allow us to adapt best to that climate. For example, in the tropics more cooling light foods such as fresh fruits and vegetables will be available. In the Arctic there will be more heavy, heat producing foods – plenty of animal products and fats. Tropical foods, if consumed in the Arctic, may even act as poison, as they contain the elements which the body requires for coping with extreme heat. Similarly, if large amounts of animal fats are consumed in the tropics, the digestive system will surely give trouble as the body does not require them or know how to utilize them.

In hot climates, grains and legumes are used as the staple food to provide sufficient protein and carbohydrate, then fruits and vegetables are added to complete the nutritional requirements.

In cold climates, however, many people find it difficult to eat grains and lentils in a sufficient quantity to supply all their protein needs. They usually feel a need for something heavier, which can be met by taking more dairy products, eggs and nuts.

- *Season*: During summer certain foods may make the body too hot, but if used in winter, these same foods may maintain the body heat at just the right level. In the extreme summer heat of India a light diet is needed. Cold weather increases the food requirement as we need to heat the body. This means that heavier and more nourishing foods should be eaten.
- *Personality type* also governs dietary needs: for example, a hot-tempered person should take more cooling foods and avoid those which increase heat and passion.

The ayurvedic texts give extensive advice for maintaining a sattwic diet based on the Indian climate, the six divisions of the year and the foods available in India.

1. *Hemant* (winter – 15th November to 15th January). Kapha (phlegm) is aggravated by cold and the following are recommended – sour, fat and salt sauces, milk preparations, sweets, fats, oils, new rice and hot liquids.
2. *Shirsha* (season of dew – 15th January to 15th March). Vata (wind) is aggravated and one should avoid pungent cold food and drink.
3. *Vasanta* (spring – 15th March to 15th May). Accumulated kapha can provoke many diseases and this can be remedied by emetics (such as kunjal) and the avoidance of heavy, sour, oily and sweet food. Barley and wheat are recommended.

4. *Grishma* (summer – 15th May to 15th July). Pitta (bile) predominates and one is advised to take tasty, cold, fluid, oily things. Avoid salt, sour, pungent and hot foods.
5. *Varsha* (rainy season – 15th July to 15th September). Vata predominates and the digestion is particularly weak. Barley, wheat, and fermented rice, boiled sauce, honey, rainwater or boiled water are recommended.
6. *Sharad* (autumn – 15th September to 15th November). Pitta predominates and one should eat a moderate quantity of sweet, light, cold foods. Rice, barley and wheat should be taken. Pure water should be obtained from a well or spring. Bitter foods and drinks, ghee, fat and oil should be avoided.

These basic recommendations have to be modified according to the temperament and constitution of the individual. For example, a person who has a predominantly vata constitution should eat those foods which do not produce wind in every season. The same applies to kapha and pitta. People who always practise meditation tend to develop excess vata and can therefore use milk, a rajasic and kapha-producing food for balance.

A person's work determines their diet to a large extent. Karma yogis who perform heavy physical work can digest any food, even meat. Heavy foods, however, would be poisonous to the jnani who sits and meditates each day. The same principle applies to the labourer and the sedentary worker. Suitable food must be selected, otherwise our system will be upset.

The tantric way

The beauty of tantra is that it accepts everything. Tantra says: enjoy what you have without becoming attached to any one way that you think is right, rather experience all and fulfil your desires. If you eat meat, enjoy it. If you eat rich, fatty foods and enjoy them, then continue. It is better to do this than to suppress your desires. The only thing that tantra suggests is that you remain aware of what you are doing. Watch what is happening to your body and mind when you eat meat, rich foods or when you eat excessively. See what is actually going on and experience all there is to experience, good and bad. Then you will know for yourself what is the right thing to eat and no neurosis or misunderstanding will arise.

7

Digestive Prana

Prana is the energy, gross and subtle, which pervades the whole cosmos. It vibrates through all life from the earth and flowers to human beings, from the tiniest atom to the largest galaxy. It is through manipulation of the mind and the pranic body that yoga can so effectively remove digestive problems. Yogic physiology transcends the physical body and puts it into its correct perspective in relation to prana, the mind and spirit.

Beyond the food body

According to the ancient yogic texts, annamaya kosha, the 'food' or physical body depends on grosser forms of prana in the form of food, water and air. It is also dependent on subtler forms of energy from the other bodies: pranamaya kosha – energy body, manomaya kosha – mental body, vijnanamaya kosha – psychic body, and anandamaya kosha – bliss body. Each subtler body gives energy to the body beneath it, thus the pranic body infuses energy into the physical body.

This energy can be divided into five main pranas according to location and function – apana, samana, prana, udana and vyana. Of these, the two mainly concerned with digestion are samana and apana.

1. *Samana* (from the navel to the diaphragm) activates and controls the digestive system – stomach, liver, pancreas

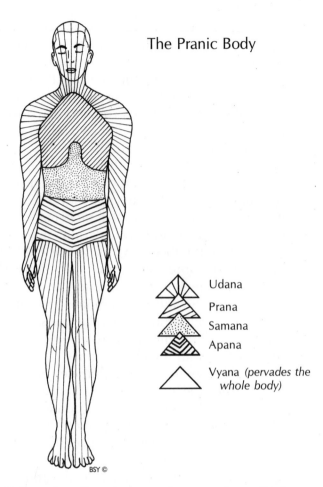

The Pranic Body

Udana

Prana

Samana

Apana

Vyana *(pervades the whole body)*

BSY ©

and small intestine. It promotes the secretion of juices
and the assimilation of nutrients. Samana is the force or
energy which prepares the rasa (essence) or juice of food
and distributes it to its respective place in the body, for
example, to the nervous system, brain, heart, etc. via the
bloodstream. The water element is said to predominate
in samana, which tends to make it white in colour and
light and cool in nature. Samana therefore mixes liquid
into the digesting food and depending on the nature of
each liquid the quality of the interaction is determined.

Samana (at the pranic level) combined with bile (at the physical level) produces heat; samana and mucus produces cooling. These two combinations work together in balancing digestion and the gastric fire which should neither overheat lest ulcer or diarrhoea form, nor should it go cold, producing such conditions as asthma. Samana also regulates the spleen, kidney and urinary process. It is a finer force than apana.

2. *Apana* (below the navel) throws out impurities via the process of elimination and expulsion. The earth element predominates and thus apana is characterized by heaviness and a downward movement. It results in defecation, urination, ejaculation, menstruation and expulsion of the foetus. Apana aids the flow of digestive juices in the intestines and pulls undigested matter towards the anus in the same way as a magnet attracts iron. Apana also aids in locomotion from the hips to the toes. The colour of apana is yellow or smoky.

In terms of digestion, these two aspects of energy function in coordination with the other pranas:

3. *Prana* (diaphragm to throat) creates hunger and thirst, moves from the mouth to the stomach and maintains body heat. The fire element is dominant, giving it the colour of gold and an upward movement.

4. *Udana* (throat and above) functions in the processes of vomiting and belching, and is the upward force that keeps the body upright. Associated with air, it is said to be blue-green in colour.

5. *Vyana* (whole body) keeps the sensory nerves active, thus helping us to perceive and taste. It aids circulation of nutrients in the blood, lymph, etc. and performs all functions of the body. Associated with ether, it is visualized as sky-blue in colour.

As well as the major divisions of prana, there are also the sub-pranas:

1. *Devadatta* (nostrils) – yawning
2. *Krikara* (throat) – sneezing, hunger and thirst

3. *Kurma* (eyelids) – winking, eyelid movement
4. *Naga* (mouth) – belching and hiccuping
5. *Dhananjaya* (whole body) – swelling, movement, nourishment and warmth.

Good digestion depends on a well balanced body and mind. One of the best ways to achieve this is through awareness and regulation of the pranas.

Cycles of prana

Food must be taken into the body at times when samana and apana are working best. Most forces of the body work in diurnal (daily) cycles, peaking and ebbing at certain times. Meals must be eaten within natural and harmonious times of body function. Most people, however, being unaware of their inner cycle, do not understand this. Thus they eat at any time, according to social convention rather than in accordance with the dictates of nature.

According to the school of thought of acupuncture, the following periods of maximal functioning of the body organs occur as follows:

Lungs	3–5 am		Bladder	3–5 pm
Large intestine	5–7 am		Kidneys	5–7 pm
Stomach	7–9 am		Heating components	7–9 pm
Spleen	9–11 am		Metabolic processes	9–11 pm
Heart	11 am–1 pm		Gall bladder	11 pm–1 am
Small intestine	1–3 pm		Liver	1–3 am

This list represents the times when prana is maximal in the organs. The opposite time represents the lowest pranic content. We can see from this that there are certain times when digestion will be easiest. The stomach is most receptive to food in the morning and least receptive in the evening. Thus the morning meals should be taken some time between 7 and 11 a.m. for the best digestion. In this way food will reach the small intestine at the best time for absorption of digested food, from 1 to 3 p.m. The morning meal should therefore be the largest as it fuels us with energy for the busy day.

The evening meal should be light and taken before sunset. As the low point of stomach prana is around 8 p.m., large meals taken at this time cannot be properly digested. Unfortunately, in many parts of the world people take their main meal between 7 and 11 p.m. and then sleep soon afterwards. This habit is detrimental to health and maybe one of the most important reasons for much of the digestive trouble facing us today. At least four hours should pass between each meal and sleep so that the little digestive fire present can adequately start off the processes of digestion. It is healthier to eat the main meal before mid-day as food is not required while sleeping.

By eating only at the correct times we flow with the natural body energies. If we take food when the pranic level is high, digestion is carried out with maximum efficiency. In this way neither energy nor nutrition are wasted and health is maintained. By eating at the wrong time, however, we swim against the current and pave the way for disease.

The nadis
In order to better understand the cycles of prana, it is necessary to gain an accurate knowledge of the nadis, the pathways of prana. This will help to regulate digestion. The three most important nadis or nerve channels in the pranic body are ida, pingala and sushumna. Sushumna flows up the centre of the spinal cord and ida and pingala wind around it in opposite directions. At the intersections of these three nadis, whirling vortices of energy called *chakras* manifest

Ida represents the parasympathetic nervous system; the passive, introvert and mental aspect. It emanates from the left side of mooladhara and is dominant when the breath is flowing through the left nostril. *Pingala* represents the sympathetic nervous system; the active, extrovert and physical aspect. It is dominant when the breath is flowing

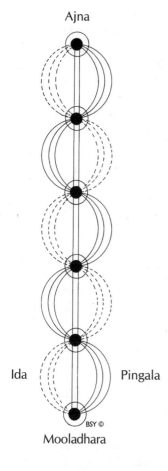

Ajna

Ida

Pingala

Mooladhara

BSY ©

through the right nostril. *Sushumna* represents the fusion of mind and body, the state of equilibrium that occurs when both nostrils are flowing.

The flow of prana in the body works in approximately 90-minute cycles, alternating between ida and pingala and spending a few moments in sushumna at the point of crossover. This science of internal rhythms, called *swara yoga*, can be applied to all the strata and phases of life. When we eat, for example, pingala nadi in the right nostril should be open. Body energy, extroversion, receptivity to external stimuli, etc. should be maximized in order to optimize the digestive process. In this way, body heat, the digestive fire and metabolism are prepared to properly 'cook' the food in the stomach and upper intestines, making it ready for absorption. Preparation of food in the stomach and upper digestive tract takes approximately 90 minutes, the time that pingala is open. After this, ida nadi opens in accordance with the natural flow of cycles. Mental energy and introversion then increase while the food is actually being absorbed into the body.

Many people believe that ida, which governs the parasympathetic nervous system, should be operational while we eat. However, if we eat while the left nostril is open, food is hurried through the intestines by increased peristalsis that results and does not have time to properly digest. Diarrhoea can result, as is the case in 'nervous diarrhoea'.

Many yogic authorities state that even when the right nostril is open and the sympathetic, stress-coping mechanism is operational, if the mind is relaxed and engaged in a pleasurable activity, this is the ideal situation. Tension is not demanding energy for its release. As the sympathetic system is conserving energy the other aspects of its dynamic nature such as the positive link with manipura chakra can manifest and the energy is then utilized for natural and creative body processes such as digestion. Health is enhanced by the proper functioning of the digestive process in harmony with the rest of the body's cycles.

Stanley Friedman of the Mt Sinai School of Medicine, USA, has postulated that stress disturbs this 90 minute cycle (called ultradian in scientific terminology) and that this disturbance desynchronizes the body.[1] As a result, psychosomatic illness can manifest because of erratic hormonal output and activity in the central and autonomic nervous systems. He has gained preliminary evidence in neurodermatitis, pointing out the necessity for harmony and balance in all bodily cycles if we are to remain healthy.

Manipura chakra

The pranic body can be energized by concentration on the chakras, especially mooladhara and manipura. This is because they represent the intersection of all the subtler bodies and therefore their manipulation, when performed correctly under proper guidance, can release large amounts of energy as well as rebalance function and even structure.

Digestion is governed by manipura chakra, the home of prana, situated in the spinal cord behind the navel. This psychic centre is concerned with the fire of the body, which is used in digestion and metabolism of food; it coordinates the nerves of the stomach, intestines and other abdominal organs. Manipura is symbolized by the sun and physiologically it is associated with the solar plexus.

This ten-petalled chakra is bright yellow in colour. The seed mantra is *ram*. Its symbolic animal is the ram, a fiery aggressive animal, and its weapon is the thunderbolt, symbolic of power and energy. When manipura is awakened the following powers are said to manifest: the ability to find hidden treasure, freedom from the fear of fire, knowledge of one's own body and the means to control it, and freedom from disease.

When manipura is weak the digestive system is sluggish, blocked or unbalanced. The digestive fire, dependent on a supply of prana from manipura, becomes less intense because it has less energy to function. Through yogic sadhana, manipura chakra is activated. The oven gets hotter and food is digested better and more quickly. This sun-like fire burns up all the toxins of the body and eliminates indigestion. It is said that a person with a fully awakened manipura can digest anything.

The power of manipura chakra is fully illustrated by the story of the great sage Agastya, who lived many thousands of years ago. Agastya once visited a demon named Atapi and his brother Vatapi. These two enjoyed disposing of their guests in a most extraordinary way. Atapi would magically turn Vatapi into a goat, which he then prepared and served to his guests. The meal finished, Atapi would call his brother forth, saying, "Vatapi, come out!" thereby killing the victim as Vatapi burst out of his stomach.

Agastya enjoyed the feast and when he had finished the meal, sat back well satisfied and patted his stomach. Atapi thought this was an opportune moment and called his brother forth, but Agastya said, "Vatapi, stay where you are! It is better for everyone if I digest you in my stomach." Agastya is also reputed to have drunk the entire ocean and is so famous for his digestive capacity that the following mantra is used to stimulate the digestive fire:

Agastyam kumbhakaranam cha shamincha vaadavaanalam
Bhojanam pachanaarthaaya smaredabhyaam cha panchakam

Loss of prana

We all know that after an excessively large meal we feel heaviness in the abdomen and lethargy throughout the whole body. Overloading the stomach and intestines results in loss of energy rather than gain. Blood is redirected from the brain and other organs to aid in the process of digestion, leaving most of the body with only the minimum supply of oxygen and nutrients. Blood is required to carry the absorbed products from the intestines to feed the cells of the body, but if it is concentrated in the digestive system for too long then the rest of the body suffers.

A light meal of grains or vegetables usually remains in the stomach for about two hours, while a fatty meal may stay in the stomach for six hours or more and its passage through the rest of the digestive tract may take a full 24 or even 36 hours. All this time the body continues working hard to digest the food, expending energy even when the peak time for digestion is well past.

Eating the wrong sort of food leads to over-secretion of one type of digestive juice, which creates imbalance in the whole digestive tract. For example, too much sugar results in excessive secretion of mucus and as a result the digestive fire is cooled, weakened, and the body becomes dull, tamasic and prone to disease. Hot, spicy, oily foods result in excessive secretion of bile, which leads to indigestion.

Depression, fear and worry automatically lower the level of one's prana. Moreover, these mental states reflect into the physical body and disturb the digestive process. Constant worry and anxiety produce gas and excessive acid secretion which leads to ulcers. An anxious person or someone burdened with a heavy load cannot enjoy their meal and this loss of satisfaction also lowers prana.

Increasing prana

A simple vegetarian diet is sufficient for the body's physical needs and keeps the pranic level high. Eating with the hands rather than with forks and spoons also increases prana. The palms and fingers radiate large amounts of prana. This fact has been substantiated by Kirlian photographs which show flames of energy shooting out of the fingertips. The hands are also an extension of the heart, a sensitive means of externalizing and expressing our inner nature. It is through the hands that psychic healers transfer prana to a diseased part of the body in order to regenerate and heal the tissues.

When we handle food, we infuse it with subtle energy. The use of spoons, knives and forks blocks this energy transfer. Taking food to the mouth with the hand is a natural way of closing a circuit of energy. When the circle closes, energy flowing out from the hands is directed back into our being through the mouth. When we touch the fingers to the lips we are performing a mudra, a gesture that reflects a psychic attitude. When we use a fork or spoon we cannot close this circuit and therefore prana is lost.

Another way to increase prana is to take meals in a happy relaxed atmosphere. Prana flows best when we are relaxed. Kirlian photographs show us that the aura of a relaxed person is stable and even, usually blue and white in colour. A tense person has an uneven, spiky emanation of smaller diameter, usually red in colour and often associated with disease.

Preparation of food is also important. When one purchases and cooks food with awareness and care, prana is transmitted into the preparation. You can actually taste it. After a meal that is well prepared and served with goodwill one feels more alive and energized.

Probably the best way to generate prana and maintain a high level of subtle energy is the regular practice of yogic techniques. The cleansing practices and asanas tone all the digestive organs, while meditation harmonizes the body with the mind. As imbalance and disturbances are gradually eliminated the appetite becomes regulated to the body's needs. When we eat in response to a healthy appetite the tendency to overeat or undereat is also reduced. Yoga synchronizes our energies and brings about a state of optimum digestive functioning.

Many spiritual aspirants regard the taking of food as a sacrament. In India, for example, the stomach is thought of as the *havan,* sacrificial fire, and food as the offering. In many homes the following verse from the *Bhagavad Gita* (4:24) is recited before every meal:

Brahman is the oblation, Brahman is the clarified butter.
By Brahman is the oblation poured into the fire of Brahman.
Brahman verily shall be reached by he who always sees Brahman
in action.

Those who take food with this attitude will increase their digestive prana and will not suffer from indigestion and other digestive disorders.

8

Fasting

Fasting is a completely natural process which each one of us does at night while we sleep, and the next morning we break our fast with breakfast. In India, many Hindus, especially ladies, practise regular fasting as part of their religious customs. Sometimes they fast once a week or on full moon days. If not a complete fast, they may take only fruits and other light foodstuffs. Fasting is also an integral part of the Muslim faith, with daylight fasting during the holy month of Ramadan. In Buddhism and Christianity fasting is also of great importance. Christ and Buddha both fasted for 40 days before reaching enlightenment and starting their missions.

Saints of every order have used fasting with prayer or meditation to reach higher spiritual states. Other people have used fasting solely as a practice to improve physical and mental health, while natural therapists have suggested that fasting is at the basis of curing many diseases. Fasting combined with yogic practices has been found to be very useful for digestive problems, helping to eliminate even long-standing conditions such as amoebic dysentery.

What is fasting?
The word fasting comes from the old English word 'fasten', meaning to fix or make firm. Under no circumstances does fasting mean starvation. In effect, the point where the body

59

starts to starve because it has depleted its nutritional reserves is the end of the fast. From the outset it is important to realize that the fasting stage only takes place so long as the body can support itself on the stored reserves within the body. Starvation begins when the body's reserves are depleted or are at a dangerously low level.

Fasting, like all other natural cures, is based on the principle that the body itself contains the most efficient healing agents. These agents are most effective when they are unhampered by the process of digestion and assimilation which tends to drain off much of the body's energies. Fasting gives these systems a much needed rest and releases energy for the elimination of toxins and for restoring the body to health.

In the optimum state of health there is no need to fast, however this is rarely the case. Most people continually overtax the body by eating too much, drinking too much and living in a continual state of tension. Instead of an adequate supply of natural nutrients, the body often receives a mixture of denatured and devitalized foodstuffs which tend to clog it up. Bodily efficiency is continually impaired by the surplus of food which it is unable to use up or throw off. Fasting gives the body time for thorough cleansing and expulsion of accumulated wastes.

In the digestive tract there is a continuous build-up of waste material such as undigested or partially digested food particles, bacteria and so on. If a person habitually overeats or suffers from constipation, this build-up will be greatly increased. This is the breeding ground for many more serious illnesses as well as general ill-health. The simplest way to clean out the whole digestive system is to miss a few meals. When no food is being ingested the body can concentrate fully on what is already there. The build-up of waste material is more effectively expelled via the bowels, kidneys and skin, bringing about a marked purification of the blood. This in turn gives a wonderful feeling of lightness and freshness.

Many people are afraid to miss even one meal, as they believe that this will weaken them. The fact is however, that Western people today suffer mainly from diseases of excess (obesity, diabetes, heart disease, etc.). They dig their grave with their teeth. Life insurance statistics reveal that a trim body is conducive to a longer life span.

Fasting and disease

Have you ever observed an animal, such as your pet dog or cat, when it is not feeling well? In most cases it will try to go somewhere where it will not be disturbed, lie down and take a complete rest. Even if you give it food it will refuse to eat. Human beings, however, find it very difficult to rest and recuperate, and for most fasting is nearly impossible. Many people think that energy comes from food and so tasty dishes are prepared for the sick person to induce him to eat. This attitude fails to take into account the fact that one of the first signs of sickness is a loss of appetite, a natural warning designed to help nature's repair work.

When bacteria invade the body the immune system is mobilized. All available energy is required and therefore physical activity should be avoided. Eating requires a lot of metabolic energy and this energy must be kept in reserve for fighting the disease. Fasting speeds up the catabolic (breakdown) process which occurs in illness, thereby helping to eliminate toxins. This appears to be the opposite view to that proposed by medical science, which offers drugs and chemicals to reduce discomfort and suppress symptoms. However, if we allow the disease to complete its natural course, it will be finished and the body will be purified. Many poisons are thrown out through the skin via perspiration and through the blood via urine. Taking food is said to allow poisons to be reabsorbed back into the body, as eating food stops catabolism and starts anabolism, the build up of the body.

Fasting is more important for those who have been on a high meat diet. Those who only take animal products such as cheese, milk and eggs require less fasting. For vegans, people on a pure vegetarian diet, fasting is not necessary, but it can be used occasionally in disease to rest the body, or to increase the digestive fire.

To claim that fasting is a 'cure-all' no matter what the nature or duration of the disease, would be foolish. Fasting is a science and it must be practised under expert guidance, especially when utilized as a therapeutic technique. The age of the sufferer, the nature of the complaint (whether acute or chronic) and various other considerations will all have to be taken into account. If an organ is structurally defective, fasting is a simple, direct and effective method of cure. It attacks disease at the roots by expelling poisons and also by increasing willpower and inducing a relaxed, meditative state of mind, which is very important in the removal of the tensions that cause disease.

Psychology of fasting

Fasting must be practised under the right circumstances and in the right frame of mind. If one is worried about toxins building up in the body or about becoming too fat, then the fast will be ineffectual. There will be tension instead of complete rest and relaxation. Such fasting is not natural; it arises out of desire or fear rather than need and throws the body's metabolism out of balance. It is better to call this sort of process starvation instead of fasting.

You will know intuitively when it is the right time to fast. Something inside says it is better to miss a meal or two. Perhaps hunger is absent or you feel that you may be getting sick. When the body tells us, "No more food, please", it is nature's signal to fast and the process feels good.

Self-imposed fasting can also be used as a meditative sadhana. If the hunger is great, you can practise antar mouna and observe everything that goes on in the body and mind. Through this you will learn many things about yourself and the importance of food in your life. You will see the psychological pull that hunger and taste exert as well as

62

your habitual approach and attitude towards food. This is a method not only to discover the inner workings of the body and mind but also to develop mental strength and willpower.

Fasting, when approached correctly, is very relaxing. As the body slows down the mind does also and this can be felt in the following ways:

- Breathing is freer
- There is greater ease of movement
- That 'tired' feeling disappears
- Fullness and discomfort in the abdomen are soon replaced by lightness
- Blood pressure is lowered

How to fast

Preparation for a fast is very important. It is not advisable to make an abrupt transition from your usual diet unless you are very ill. In this case all solid food should be eliminated from your diet and plenty of fluids consumed so as to flush the kidneys. If you are well and able to prepare for the fast, first abstain from meat and heavy foods, then over the next few days switch over to a light fruit diet. After this you can commence the fast.

The following suggestions will help to make your fast more successful:

1. If possible, fasting should be undertaken during the warmer periods of the year. During cold weather food is converted into energy to keep the body warm. Fasting at this time makes the body more susceptible to cold. Of course, in the case of acute disease a fast can still be undertaken, but the house should be kept warm and whenever you go outside be sure to wear plenty of warm clothing.
2. Few people are aware of the benefits of fasting, so before you begin make sure that your family and friends understand the basics of fasting and your goal. Fasting in the early stages is difficult enough without having nagging relatives trying to force food down your throat. A positive,

encouraging atmosphere amidst family and friends is most helpful. If you wish to fast for a long period of time and your surroundings are not suitable, we advise you to stay in an ashram or similar institution where fasting is regularly undertaken with the aid of expert guidance. Most people are a little uncertain during their first attempt at fasting so it is essential that the environment be as congenial as possible.

3. The body itself is the most reliable indicator of how long the fast should be. This applies whether one is fasting for cure of disease or for general cleansing. Also the severity of the disease may determine the length of the fast. As the constitution of each of us is slightly different, the duration of fasting must suit each individual. Rely on what the body tells you rather than on the experience of others.

   The duration of the fast depends largely on the purpose for which the fast is undertaken. For a general cleanout, one to three days per month is sufficient. If fasting is practised once a week the benefits will be greatly enhanced. For more specific purposes the standard duration is three days if one is without guidance. This is generally long enough to give the whole system a complete rest.

4. In a pure fast one should take only plain water, nothing else. It is good to drink plenty of water while fasting as this increases the natural process of purification. In a fast of longer than two days, one should take water with a little lemon juice (no sugar) three times daily to aid the cleansing process.

5. In a one-day fast, feelings of weakness (if they occur) are largely psychological. Your mental attitude will make all the difference. People have been known to fast for many days and grow progressively stronger. Some people say that on a one day fast it is essential to maintain all normal activities, for if one rests all day 80% of the benefits will be lost due to lack of natural blood circulation. While fasting

most people experience a wonderful feeling of freshness and lightness, and many report that they can carry out their daily duties even more efficiently. Others say we should take a complete rest. The average person may wish to avoid strenuous physical activities on a fast of two days or longer. You must find your own middle way.

6. In prolonged fasts hunger sensations disappear after the first few days even though the hunger contractions of the stomach may persist. This is thought to be due to an adaptive process in the brain. Drinking water helps to relieve the desire for food, but never drink iced water. Also use bhujangini mudra to reduce hunger. Keep in mind that there is a difference between hunger and appetite. Hunger is the natural call of the body for food in order to maintain itself, while appetite is hunger of the mind.

7. It is beneficial to take an enema or to do basti or laghoo shankhaprakshalana on the day of fasting, or the day after, especially if there is no bowel movement. Do not use laxatives.

8. Bathe once or twice a day with cold or lukewarm water. Inner and outer cleanliness go hand in hand.

9. Keep yourself occupied mentally and do not think about food. One who fasts but spends the whole time waiting for the fast to be over is wasting their time and creating mental tension.

10. Fasting is not generally advised for reducing fat. The average dieter will fast for one day and then eat enough for three days the day after.

11. Look upon fasting as a spiritual practice and when you fast never advertise it. Aside from its physical benefits, fasting is a powerful method of developing willpower and self-discipline.

12. The important thing to remember in fasting is moderation. Never fast if the cravings of the body and mind become excessive, and don't fast if you do not feel like

it. Be open to the possibility of fasting and use it when the need arises. It is said in the *Bhagavad Gita* (6:16): "Yoga is not possible for one who eats too much, or for he who abstains too much from eating."

Breaking the fast

There is a great tendency to overeat upon completion of the fast. Much care should be taken to ensure that a proper diet is followed. The method of breaking the fast will depend on the duration of the fast, but generally the first food taken should be liquid – fresh fruit juice or milk. This especially applies for fasts longer than 24 hours. Orange juice diluted with water taken every two hours is a popular way to break a fast. The first solid food to be taken should be something easy to digest, like melon or vegetable broth. Take only small amounts and chew each mouthful well.

The following diets are suggested after the liquid diet:

- *Fruit diet*: preferably composed of chopped fresh fruits in season: apples and dates or peaches and dates, for example, taken in small quantities every two or three hours.
- *Milk diet*: take a glass of milk every few hours as desired.
- *Gruel diet*: boil a teaspoon of oatmeal or barley in a pint of water and add a pinch of salt or sugar. Take small amounts at first, slowly increase over a few days.

After breaking the fast, keep the following points in mind:

- Drink plenty of water.
- Your stomach will have shrunk and will require less food so take care not to overeat.
- Do not overexercise for the first few days.

Partial fast

Many people will find it impossible or impractical to complete a prolonged fast. For them we suggest a partial fast which can give many benefits although not to the same degree as a full fast. A partial fast involves restricting the diet to fruits,

66

which cleanse the body by their accompanying laxative
influence on the bowels and also supply the blood with
needed minerals and vitamins. Here are some dietary
suggestions for carrying out a partial fast:
1. Six to eight oranges a day – one at a time every few hours.
2. One grapefruit every three or four hours.
3. A quarter of a pint of fresh fruit juice every three hours,
   up to six times a day.
4. One cupful of vegetable broth every four to six hours.

Should children fast?

Children often know instinctively when to fast. If you let a
child miss a meal or even a day's food when he is sick, for
example, and doesn't want to eat, real hunger will soon
appear. The child will naturally want food when the body
requires it, especially if snacks in between meals are stopped
and raw fruit is substituted for after dinner sweets. There
are times when the instinctive wisdom of the infant or child
in such matters may be far greater than many of us give
credit for.

Fasting sadhana

While fasting, yogic practices should be directed towards
helping to eliminate the toxins of the body. The following
techniques are particularly useful:
- *Hatha yoga shatkriya:* Laghoo shankhaprakshalana, kunjal
  and neti, basti.
- *Asana:* Pawanmuktasana, vajrasana, shavasana.
- *Pranayama:* Bhramari, nadi shodhana, ujjayi
- *Meditation:* Yoga nidra, antar mouna.

   Note: If you are fasting for illness seek competent advice
on sadhana combined with karma yoga, bhakti yoga and
jnana yoga for faster, deeper and more long-term results.

9

Am I Hungry!

Hunger implies emptiness and the desire to find fullness, not only on the physical level but on the emotional, mental and spiritual levels as well. Hunger commences when we are only a few hours out of the womb. We experience separation from our source, our mother, and hunger for her food and her comforting presence. Hunger originates in the search for fulfilment, happiness and completion, but in the outside world it takes many forms. Some seek to satisfy it through food, others through work, sports or leisure. Whatever external activity is performed, it has at its base the deep hunger for reunion with the higher self, for the return to our true nature, peace and bliss. It is a hunger for the permanent cessation of all hunger.

Physical hunger

Hunger is a sign of good health and its absence a symptom of disease, particularly of the gastrointestinal tract. Hunger signals the brain that food is required. It has three components:

1. *Appetite* refers to food preference, which the physiologist Cannon has summarized as that which "arises from the experience of previous pleasures; a wishing, longing or yearning for something especially desirable". We are hungry for those things we like and their very thought, sight, smell or taste elicits copious secretions of saliva

and gastric juice, whereas just the opposite occurs for those things we do not like. When the sense of smell is destroyed, the appetite is reduced or lost. Genetic factors also appear to play a part, for example, lions do not eat bananas and monkeys do not eat meat. Appetite, therefore, determines what we eat. It is linked to swadhisthana chakra, the pleasure centre.

2. *Hunger pangs* determine when and how much we eat. They are commonly described as a disagreeable ache or gnawing sensation in the upper central abdomen. They are believed by some to be caused by contractions of the empty stomach although this has not yet been proved. The point at which hunger is satisfied by taking food into the body depends to a large extent on social customs and appetite. This aspect of hunger is related to manipura chakra and the digestive fire.

3. *Hunger drive* is said to be a deeper phenomenon than hunger pangs, and may be instinctive. Some authorities say that it results from cellular consciousness seeking to replenish a diminishing nutritional supply. It appears to be linked with energy expenditure, the body demanding food for survival, perhaps at subconscious or unconscious levels. It still exists even when the nervous connections from the stomach to the brain are cut and the contractions of the stomach associated with hunger pangs cease. It is also present when the stomach is cut out. This deep hunger drive appears to be linked with mooladhara chakra, the centre for self-preservation.

These three factors work concurrently, creating a deep urge to eat, to take in nourishment, to survive. This signals the brain and stimulates the stomach to contract, causing the feeling of gnawing emptiness called 'hunger'. This feeling is strongest on an empty stomach and disappears with the ingestion of food. It is temporarily stopped by sham chewing or swallowing, smoking and drinking alcohol, and also by tightening the belt. Strong emotions also quickly abolish it. Appetite determines what we eat to tone down the hunger, but this is often influenced by other factors. For example, sexual suppression leads many people to overeat sweet foods.

Within us the mechanisms exist which tell us exactly how much we need to eat and when to stop. Rats who eat a diet diluted with cellulose or kaolin, indigestible substances, will increase their intake to maintain a constant caloric intake and weight.[1] A dehydrated dog will at once replace its fluid loss up to the threshold or diuresis (loss through the kidneys).[2] Therefore, the body appears to be able to sensitively and accurately measure its intake. This has two apparent stages – the first is a temporary one, perhaps mediated by the psychological satisfaction of taking in, and the second is the permanent phase of satiation registered by the satiety centre in the hypothalamus.

Awareness is an important factor in separating physical hunger from mental hunger. By developing awareness we can become sensitive to our inner body signals and needs, then we can avoid overindulgence by stopping at the point of satiation and eating for the body and not for the mind. For some people this may require patience and mindfulness as food habits are not so easy to change. However, this is an excellent means of eradicating such conditions as obesity, dyspepsia and other digestive problems which often arise because of habitual overindulgence. Awareness is the key to controlling hunger.

Mental hunger

When you desire something and think about it for some time, it becomes a mental hunger or a craving. Such hunger is more than just the need for food, it is the desire to fill in the vacuum which we have created in our lives. Craving is an unconscious mechanism to compensate for deep insecurity, to satisfy the desire for sensual pleasure, or to compensate for lack of power or unrequited love.

When we crave, we approach the world from a sense of self-centredness. We are aware of the things in the world purely from our own subjective point of view. It is obvious that this approach is totally unrealistic and if we take it to its logical conclusion, it can only end in suffering through the frustration of our desires. Tension is thus produced and the body becomes unbalanced, diseased, weak and prone to indigestion.

The obvious antidote to this form of suffering is to try to attain a more selfless, objective view. Yoga and a meditative attitude of awareness will help to accomplish this. Instead of seeing everything with an attitude of grasping and taking, we learn to give, and find that only in this way can we truly gain. Then our hunger is satisfied and we turn inwards in our search for fulfilment, rather than outwards.

The yogic approach

In yogic terminology, when hunger is tainted with desire, it is called a *klesha*. The five kleshas are the root of all suffering and pain. In Patanjali's *Yoga Sutras* (2:3) it states: "Ignorance, I feeling (ego), liking (desire), disliking (aversion) and fear of death are the pains."

The objects of pleasure cause the mind to run after them. When we overindulge in pleasure we suffer disease. This is a universal law that binds us to the lower levels of consciousness. For example, if we overeat we suffer from indigestion. Pleasure and pain originate in ignorance (*avidya*), and they are the prime motivating forces in human beings, existing at the roots of our being.

Most people eat as soon as they feel the slightest hunger in an effort to avoid pain. A yogi, however, has developed the willpower to feel hunger without having to satisfy it immediately. He awaits and allows the digestive fire to increase and when he is really hungry he eats. The yogi is aware of hunger pangs, but like all sensations he sees their temporary nature and never allows them to control him. He sees hunger as a healthy form of suffering, far better than the suffering which results from overindulgence, and with this mental attitude he can actually enjoy his experience of hunger.

71

The yogi eats neither out of boredom nor as a compulsive and repetitive habit. He eats to live and does not live to eat. At a certain level of yogic achievement, hunger ceases completely and even food is not required to maintain the body. This occurs when the individual consciousness has merged with the supreme. It is fulfilment of hunger at the spiritual level.

Bow and arrow technique

Before reaching this stage, however, the yogi must first become aware of physical hunger and see how it affects the body/mind. Then he can transmute and sublimate his hunger for worldly things into a hunger, a deep desire for spiritual life and inner knowledge. A good exercise for this is the bow and arrow technique which stretches our desire to the limit, thereby forcing us to break through into hitherto unexplored realms. By using the things of the world we can effectively eliminate their influence on us in the same way as we use a thorn to remove a thorn. The method is that of alternating attachment and detachment.

• *Phase 1: The drawing of the bow.* Initially we try to detach ourselves from the things we like or desire or crave. Depending on the environment this is practised in, and on the guru, as much as possible of the variety and spice are removed from the diet. For a period of one to three months, we exist on a monotonous diet. In this time many desires, cravings, thoughts of all descriptions and excuses to break the discipline will arise. If we manage to last the time allotted, however, we will experience many new feelings and states of consciousness. During this time the practice of antar mouna is used to allow the impurities of the mind to surface and be eliminated without our involvement.

• *Phase 2: Releasing the arrow.* When the allotted time is over, we feast to our heart's content on all those things we have been craving. This indulgence is harmless, even if it does cause a little digestive upset for a day or two afterwards. During this indulgence we really enjoy the objects of craving and at the same time we usually find that these things are not actually worth the time and energy we spent craving for them. In this phase we experience the futility of trying to satisfy the senses through the sense objects. Satisfaction is not to be found in this sort of activity. One experience of this kind is usually enough to start off a chain reaction and prompt us to search for higher spiritual things. Thus drawing the bow and releasing the arrow leads automatically to the next phase.

- *Phase 3: Striking the target.* We may not hit the bull's eye and reach the ultimate desire-free state the first time but at least our consciousness has been turned in the right direction. We have at least set our aim towards the higher goal. During this phase a guru is necessary to steer us clear of the pitfalls and to aim our arrow towards the right target. He provides us with the light by which to aim our shots and gives techniques to smooth our journey. In this way we gradually eliminate our gross desires and purify our minds.

If you want to try this technique for yourself, start by cutting down on all snacks, sweets and highly processed foods. Take only two simple meals each day, consisting of three or four basic items which are not changed from meal to meal. If this is too difficult then stop all food and drink with sugar for a week to a month or stop all salt. If you lack the discipline for this also then the ashram environment is the best alternative.

Hunger sadhana

In order to achieve an objective balanced view of hunger, it is necessary to become progressively less involved and entangled with habitual cravings and desires. This can best be achieved gradually with the help of yogic techniques.

1. **For decreasing hunger** probably the best technique is bhujangini mudra in which air is taken into the stomach

until it is completely full, and then the air is belched out. This reduces the feeling of emptiness within by stimulating the satiety centre in the brain. Use it any time you feel hunger coming on and try to limit your food intake in this way. Other useful techniques include:

- *Asana*: Vajrasana (before meals), shavasana (with breath awareness), shashankasana.
- *Pranayama*: Nadi shodhana, bhramari, seetkari.
- *Meditation*: Any meditation technique, but especially antar mouna.

2. **For increasing hunger** the best techniques are:
- *Hatha yoga shatkriya:* Shankhaprakshalana, kunjal and neti, agnisar, nauli.
- *Asana:* Pawanmuktasana part 2, surya namaskara, paschimottanasana, bhujangasana, shalabhasana, dhanurasana, ardha matsyendrasana, sarvangasana.
- *Pranayama:* Bhastrika, ujjayi.
- *Mudra:* Tadagi mudra.

Karma yoga is one of the best ways to increase the digestive fire, especially if it takes the form of hard physical work. Bhakti yoga also increases the hunger, especially for spiritual things. Jnana yoga reduces physical hunger by reducing the passions of the mind and yet increases spiritual hunger.

Digestive Disorders

10

From Darkness to Light

Fear of disease is one of the greatest stresses facing people in the world. Every day we see someone, perhaps a close friend or relative, stricken and suffering with a painful and long-term disease. Digestive diseases are probably the most common and irritating of all conditions because, as a rule, they are minor chronic problems which are just bad enough to intrude into our conscious awareness and to disturb the routine and joy of living. Irritating indigestion, painful piles, chronic constipation, disturbing diarrhoea or an unpleasant ulcer make our lives miserable and there is very little that we have been able to do to remove them from our lives. Now yoga is being recognized as the solution to this long-standing medical problem.

Disease arises because of weakness. In most of us this weakness is not inherent but has developed because of bad lifestyle and habits. There are many inbuilt defence mechanisms which are by nature designed to correct deficiencies and imbalances. Their function derives its power from prana, whose nature is essentially life-giving and life-enhancing. It is only when we develop neuroses at the mental level, emotional storms and passions, physical toxins and tensions, that we effectively cut ourselves off from this force and its effervescence. It is because of prana that most of us are born healthy and remain healthy for the majority of our lifespan. Our basic nature is healthy, whole, complete. However, if we try hard enough we can upset the delicate mechanisms within and cause ourselves suffering.

If we look closely at our lives we see that the disease producing process is a 24-hour affair, one that may continue even into our sleep/resting time. For example, if we really want to make ourselves sick we can sit at a desk for eight hours a day working as a clerk, typist, telephone operator or accountant. After work we may go home and sit some more, reading a book, watching television, talking to friends or occupying ourselves with some other spectator activity which does not demand our active participation. This exercise deficient life leads to obesity, constipation, haemorrhoids and other more serious diseases, including heart and circulatory conditions. Alternatively, if our job demands some degree of responsibility, such as that of a doctor, business executive or teacher, we may take our problems home with us, disturbing our sleep with our anxieties and worries. Without sufficient physical and mental rest, and peace and joy, dyspepsia and ulcers form. The disease process creeps into every aspect of our lives.

With any disease, the inner and outer world take on a strange and sometimes terrifying aspect. Fear of the unknown fills the mind and here we have one of the major mechanisms responsible for the perpetuation of ill health in our lives. If we are scared of sickness, then this fear in itself weakens the mind and body, allowing the seeds of disharmony to grow. Fear upsets the brain's controlling mechanisms and causes bodily disturbances, especially in the sympathetic nervous system and adrenal glands. At the subconscious mental level, fear colours our whole attitude to life, to our relationships with other people and with ourselves. It stems from *dwesha,* aversion to suffering, the opposite of *raga,* the desire for pleasure. We fear being hurt and this inherent survival mechanism springs up even when it is not justified. If it prevents us from living full lives, it becomes a neurotic, anxiety-producing, destructive process.

78

At the root of our fears and sufferings, imagined and otherwise, lies ignorance. We lack sufficient knowledge to counteract the processes involved in our becoming sick. Ignorance about the body, diet and other aspects of our lives leads us to make mistakes. Of course, mistakes are necessary to a degree, for without them we cannot grow and learn the lessons of life. However, with knowledge, we make fewer and less painful mistakes.

There are many diseases which bring fear to the minds of most people, and perhaps cancer and heart disease rank foremost. Many diseases seem to be incurable and appear to be able to strike at any time. It takes a lot of courage to face life and it takes even more courage to face up to our own ignorance and shortcomings. The resolute determination that grows out of courage allows us to live full lives, free from fear and disease. We must resolve to become strong, to make the mind firm, steady and unshakeable, to handle the problems of life, if we are to remove anger, frustration and other destructive emotions which eat away at the body.

Yoga is universally accepted as a system capable of calming the mind, balancing the emotions and harmonizing the body. It is a system that encourages natural energies and functions to continue in the best possible way. Yoga works with the body, not against it. Asanas massage muscles and organs so as to enhance blood flow and stimulate blocked nervous connections. Pranayama helps to regulate the metabolic processes at a cellular level and also coordinates brain function with external need. For example, ujjayi calms the energies of the mind, allows us to gain control of the automatic processes within the brain and to gain insight into life in general. In this way we overhaul the entire human vehicle and make it fit for good living.

We can understand better how yoga helps us to undo the tangle of mental and physical energies that leads to disease if we take the analogy of the bow and arrow. These tools represent the yogic techniques that enable us, if we know how, to hit the bull's eye of good health. We must first learn how to use these implements, for they are the same in everyone's hands, but everyone uses them differently. Our goal and aim must be correct and the pull on the string neither too hard nor too soft if we are to hit the target and not under or overshoot. The same applies to the yogic techniques. They are available to all and serve as channels to redirect mental and physical structure and function. However, the degree of balance with which we approach them: determination balanced with patience, power with gentleness, serious application with humour and insight, will determine the degree of success and the speed with which cure is attained.

Yoga is especially valuable in digestive disorders of all kinds, not only in the removal of existing problems but also in the prevention of recurrence. Medical science plays a vital role in acute conditions, emergencies both medical and surgical, to allay the fears that arise when the disease process appears to be getting out of hand, to relieve pain and suffering, while all the time nature does the work. However, only yoga is able to strengthen the constitutional factors in the body and remove the root cause.

Yoga also plays a vital role in removing fear, for it allows us to gain experience and begin to cure ourselves of our individual digestive ailment. Yoga is instrumental in the dawning of our own self-confidence, for it provides us with a system by which we can handle any digestive trouble as it arises. Knowledge of what to do in a situation gives us a path to follow out of the darkness and into the light. The attitude and the self-confidence derived from this knowledge generates a lot of healing energy, enough to make us feel good and to redirect the internal process from a negative fearful state to a positive creative one.

Cure is not the only aim of yoga. Once we can control the processes of the body with our awareness and mental faculties, we rediscover the amazing world within. The play of energies and the function of the various bodily organs is like a new universe, each organ representing a galaxy and the cells the myriad solar systems within it. This universe and its inherent driving power actually opens up to our inner eye. We begin to realize that within us lies an incredible force responsible for the creation of the atoms, chemicals and various other constituents of the body. A total change in consciousness takes place, simultaneously releasing a fantastic surge of energy which courses through our veins and fills us with vitality and dynamism.

This prana is the means to achieve everything that we want in life and beyond. The awakening of this energy seems to have two main stages:

1. A rebalancing stage in which an unconscious surge of energy into the body occurs. In the ashram environment, where this energy is particularly strong, we see the first signs of such a change taking on many forms. For example, it can take the form of a cleansing reaction such as loose stools, boils, colds or fevers of unexplained origin, though these are of a mild nature as a rule. A good analogy to explain this phenomenon is a strong blast of water pushing dirt and impurities out of a blocked pipe. The cleansing reaction alternates with times of vibrant good health and an overabundance of energy (when the pipe is free from impediment). Some people in this stage have so much energy that they can eat up to 15 to 20 thick rotis (the equivalent to approximately three large loaves of bread) per meal, without doing any harm to their digestive systems.

So this stage is characterized by the mental and physical energies oscillating and undulating in the same way as a boat moves up and down in rough water. It is obvious that the release of such force must take place in the presence of a skilled and experienced guru, one who can handle the turbulent and sometimes violent reactions which result from the meeting of an impure body with the pure force of prana.

2. A controlling stage in which the initially turbulent reaction is replaced by balance and equilibrium. This is the stage of control and implies the presence of awareness. In this stage the body is functioning close to optimal efficiency.

The thermostats, secretors, regulators and other tissues are all in order. Digestion is at its peak. In this state we get from one piece of bread what would previously have taken ten pieces to provide.

Yogis in this stage have been known to survive on just a glass of milk and a little fruit per day. The perfection of stage 2, which is a long and circuitous process, culminates in perfect dynamic equilibrium or samadhi. In this stage the yogi can either choose to eat as much as he wants or to subsist on absolutely no food intake. This is because his level of function has shifted out of the physical and into the more subtle body. His expanded awareness allows him to control a wider spectrum of digestive activity. However, to attain such a state requires many years of practice and guidance.

It is our hope that the following material will provide an adequate guide to good health and balance in life. The knowledge contained herein has come directly from our guru, guide and inspirer, Swami Satyananda Saraswati. It is based on many years of practical experience in helping others to help themselves and is designed to give people an understanding of their physical condition in relation to the other aspects of being. A thorough knowledge of the digestive tract and the possible problems that can arise helps to enhance our awareness. This in turn increases our ability to control the digestive tract. Control of one system quickly leads to control of all the bodily systems and deeper knowledge of the higher aspects of the self.

Using yoga we have the tools to help us increase our awareness so as to take over control of all the physical and mental processes. The benefits accrued extend into our daily life and help to raise not just our health but our whole being into the light of a higher and happier life.

11

Digestion and the Mind

Indigestion is a psychosomatic disease, which means it has its roots in the mind and manifests in the body. The link between the digestive system and the mind is easily demonstrated when we realize that if we are hungry, just the thought of food is enough to start our salivary and digestive juices running. As soon as we fill the stomach, the mind is satisfied. Mental depression produces loss of appetite accompanied by a heavy feeling in the stomach, while fear gives us butterflies, a fluttering feeling in the pit of our stomach.

The mind-body is an integrated unit so that mental conflicts are reflected physically in one way or another and vice-versa. For this reason, mental problems, whether large or small, tend to weaken the body, and the digestive system is one of the most susceptible areas. Weakness sometimes starts off as indigestion and discomfort and can quickly progress to more serious diseases.

The stomach and stress

Of all the digestive organs, the stomach is the one most often subjected to research into the effects of mind on body. As early as 1833 the physician Beaumont observed the reddening of the stomach lining during emotional upset in a patient with a gunshot wound. This wound had not healed properly but had left a fistula, a passage from the stomach to the outside, through which Beaumont made his observations and collected secretions under different emotional states including hunger, pain, frustration, anger, joy, sorrow and contentment.

More recent studies have shown that students who feel the pressures of serious examinations secrete excessive hydrochloric acid, the corrosive effect of which is probably one of the major causes of peptic ulcer.[1] These findings were confirmed in individuals in whom anxiety, anger and resentment were elicited by a stressful interview.[2]

Probably every physician and ulcer patient knows the relationship between mental tension, stress and ulcers. Ulcer is the classic example of psychosomatic disease. It is estimated that one out of ten Americans will suffer a peptic ulcer during their lifetime and most of these will be in high pressure jobs, especially executives in competitive professions such as advertising. Professions such as taxi driving, where they are subjected to constant tension, very commonly develop ulcers.

Sidney Cobb, of Brown University (USA) has determined that air traffic controllers who are under keen stress have a higher incidence of ulcers, hypertension and diabetes than do second class licensees not under comparable stress. He also found that autoworkers laid off in Detroit showed an increased incidence of ulcers at the time of their forced termination. Other workers developed cancer, arthritis, hypertension, alcoholism and gout.[3]

Neal Miller, psychologist at Rockefeller University (USA) and a pioneer in the study of the autonomic nervous system states: "There is considerable evidence that people under stress conditions, like combat, have stomach lesions. This is backed up by experimental evidence that...subjecting animals to stress will cause stomach lesions."[4] John W. Mason of the Walter Reed Army Institute of Research (USA) has been quoted as saying: "There is no shortage of data relating disease to psychological factors. The shortage is only in our knowledge of the mediating mechanisms."[5]

In this light, different mental mechanisms and examples of personality types are now being observed to try to explain the psychosomatic factor in disease. In the area of digestive problems, jealousy is thought to be an underlying cause of ulcer, anger of hyperacidity and dyspepsia, greed of obesity, frustration of diarrhoea, and possessiveness of constipation. In other disease areas such as cancer, victims are thought to be those who were not close to their parents in childhood and hide their emotions. Even when under stress they say, "Everything's fine!" Heart attack victims tend to be just the opposite as they feel they are under greater stress than they really are. People with arthritis, especially women, tend to have unfulfilled ambitions due to feelings of inadequacy when they were children. Many of these conditions set in after being triggered by some traumatic experience.

One thing that has become clearer is the fact that non-specific mental stresses are at the base of many illnesses and that much of the effect of stress is due to our inner response to it. Hans Selye in his book *Stress Without Distress* states: "We have seen that it is immaterial whether a stressor is pleasant or unpleasant; its stressor effect depends merely on the intensity of the demand made upon the adaptive capacity of the body." "Mental tensions, frustrations, insecurity and aimlessness are among the most damaging stressors and psychosomatic studies have shown how often they cause migraine headaches, peptic ulcers, heart attacks, hypertension..."

How the mind affects the body and causes disease is a matter of psyche and soma and their interrelationship. In order to remove the roots of disease, and prevent them from growing back or taking further root in some other area, we must first understand the role of thought on emotion and emotion on body.

The mind-body link

The digestive system is a very sensitive mirror of the mind because it is almost wholly under the influence of the autonomic nervous system, which in turn is thought to be governed by the limbic area of the brain. The emotions and mental processes act directly on the limbic area of the brain and via the autonomic nervous system they affect the stomach and digestive organs.

If you remove a piece of intestine from the body and place it in a supportive environment where all its relaxed needs are met, it will live and continue to contract and relax rhythmically. It acts as an independent creature in this environment, albeit a very primitive one. This is because nature has equipped it with its own intrinsic nerve supply, which causes it to beat rhythmically in the same way as the heart muscle beats, because of its inner electrical activity.

When we view this process within the context of the body, other controlling factors come into play, the major controller being the brain-mind complex. The brain sends wires (nerves) out to the periphery so that messages can pass freely. Because the digestive system is amongst the most primitive we possess, it does not require conscious control. Unconscious control is enough and this is attained through the autonomic nervous system.

The sympathetic and parasympathetic branches of the autonomic nervous system are antagonistic but complement-ary in the healthy individual. The parasympathetic system, which dominates in the relaxed state, turns on the digestive juices, speeds up peristalsis and opens the sphincters. The sympathetic system does the opposite. They are like the tone and volume controls on a radio, increasing or decreasing the volume but not altering the program.

These systems are balanced and can be thought of as two sides of the same coin. They depend on each other and must be properly harmonized to function at peak efficiency. Imbalance obviously results in disease.

In most people the control of the autonomic system is subconscious. Mental and neurological circuits, which have usually been pre-programmed either by genetics or environ-mental conditioning, operate in the main controlling

86

The Autonomic Nervous System

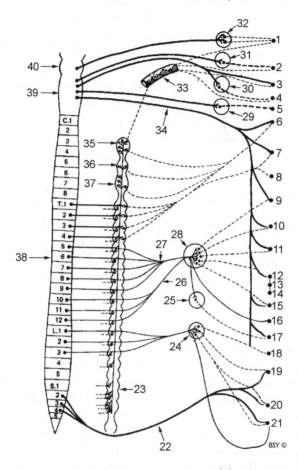

1. Eye	15. Pancreas	29. Optic ganglion
2. Lacrimal gland	16. Adrenal medulla	30. Submaxillary ganglion
3. Submaxillary gland	17. Kidney	31. Sphenopalatine ganglion
4. Sublingual gland	18. Colon	32. Ciliary ganglion
5. Parotid gland	19. Rectum	33. Carotid artery & plexus
6. Heart	20. Bladder	34. Vagus nerve
7. Larynx, trachea, bronchi	21. Sex organs	35. Superior cervical ganglion
8. Lung	22. Pelvic nerve	36. Middle cervical ganglion
9. Stomach	23. Sympathetic chain	37. Inferior cervical ganglion
10. Small intestine	24. Inferior mesenteric ganglion	38. Spinal cord
11. Abdominal blood vessels	25. Superior mesenteric glanglion	39. Medulla
12. Liver	26. Small splanchnic nerve	40. Midbrain
13. Gall bladder	27. Greater splanchnic nerve	
14. Bile ducts	28. Celiac ganglion	

mechanisms. For example, the rate of metabolism of food, energy turnover and thus degrees of hunger, appetite and frequency of food intake depend on a complex neuro-endocrine balance. The thyroid gland, for example, which controls metabolism, should not be over or underactive as this may result in abnormal physical and mental states. The circuits within the hypothalamus that control hunger and satiation, the autonomic nervous system and the endocrines must be in tune with our deeper needs.

The mind works synchronously and interdependently with the body. It acts especially on the limbic system, which contains the hypothalamus, the controller of our reactions to emotional and mental change and their resultant effects on the body. Autonomic stability therefore depends on mental and emotional stability. This stability is vital because the autonomic nervous system controls all our vital functions and mediates our involuntary responses to our environment.

The autonomic system in human beings can be either stable or labile (unstable). The labile or weak system is more prone to psychosomatic disease and mental illness. Worry, tension, dissipation of concentration, an unorganized and unfulfilling lifestyle, and an inability to cope with stress are the major factors operating in autonomic lability.

The mind is like the sea, the body is the land and their sphere of interaction is the seashore. When the mind is peaceful and relaxed, the sea is calm. However, when the mind is troubled the sea becomes turbulent and waves beat against the shore, tearing away large sections of the land. This is the psychosomatic disease process which results in indigestion, constipation, peptic ulcer, diarrhoea and so many other minor and major diseases.

The mechanisms of disease
Anxiety is known to cause all manner of gastrointestinal malfunctions, running the entire gamut from indigestion to ulceration. Why this occurs is a vexing question. Perhaps we can understand the process better if we look at primitive

animals whose nervous system is roughly equivalent to ours at the level of the autonomic nervous system, the hind or primitive brain. Some animals react to stress by evacuating the bowel, presumably to make more energy available by reducing the load the body has to carry. In some primitive creatures, notably the sea slug, the whole lower intestine is jettisoned, after which it grows back at a later date. In higher animals, such as vertebrates (animals with spinal cords), stress and anxiety may produce diarrhoea, especially in chronic states of tension when the sympathetic nervous system is fatigued.

When we are stressed the whole body is geared to reducing body weight, and definitely not to food intake. We should not eat when we are tense. This is a point that most people do not understand and because of this many people fall sick. Initially, digestive upsets, diarrhoea and constipation may occur, but later more serious diseases develop when we habitually ignore the warning signals of our body and fail to remedy stress. Our internal attitudes and external environment can create a state of ongoing stress which is difficult to remedy unless we have a system like yoga. If we are in a stressful state in which the tendency is to evacuate the gastrointestinal contents but we persist in eating, a great deal of harm is done. However, this is a common state of affairs in our modern world. Many business people have lunch in a stressed state, anxious to get a large account or contract from an important client, hurrying their food, all the while stressed by their ambitions and desires.

When the stressful state becomes ongoing and inappropriate, the different parts of the gastrointestinal tract start to work independently of each other. Communication breaks down between cells, organs and their various functions. The stomach may secrete too much acid while the intestines secrete too little of something else. Inability to digest results and we lose touch with our body.

Some animals have evolved mechanisms to adapt to stress. For example, rabbits and other ruminants have developed a stomach in which they can deposit grass. While eating in an open sunny area, exposed to predators, the animal must be continually alert and excited so as to be prepared to flee at the slightest warning signal. Later, when the animal is safe in the cool protection of dappled shade or its burrow, it can regurgitate the rumen and chew carefully and thoroughly, enjoying food as it should be enjoyed. Human beings have no such mechanism, however, and must rely on external methods such as yoga to induce a relaxed and controlled state of mind, even in the midst of stress such as the business lunch, and thereby regain control of his inner world.

Calming the sea

Yoga is probably the best way to calm the stormy, turbulent mind that eats away the body in the psychosomatic process. Yoga is a wellknown antidote for anxiety, tension and worry as it aids the natural, internal processes and mechanisms of the body to function more effectively. It accomplishes this through its relaxing and soothing action on the mind and body. The lower, more primitive parts of the brain such as the autonomic nervous system and hypothalamus are rebalanced and integrated with the higher nervous system. It is important to know and remember this, because if we do not find a remedy for stress we are likely to suffer from all sorts of psychosomatic, degenerative and organic diseases.

In the short term, asana and pranayama are utilized to rejuvenate and manipulate the physical body and this has a soothing effect on the mind. When we make the body stronger we also strengthen the mind. In the long term we need to utilize a variety of simple techniques to reintegrate the lost functions of the body and mind into our conscious awareness. Meditation and concentration exercises achieve this.

By awareness and the practice of relaxation, we can control our bodies and manipulate them as desired. If we are in a stressful situation, our awareness warns us not to eat but to relax with breath awareness or some meditative technique. When we practise these techniques regularly as a part of our daily lives, we relax spontaneously and naturally. As our insight, understanding and intuition are developed, fears and ignorance which lead to tension are removed. Until this stage occurs, inculcate awareness through the medium of yoga, so that you can develop the ability to know when you are tense and when you are relaxed. Only then will you enjoy food the way it should be enjoyed and with it vibrant good health.

12

Pass the Antacid, Please

Do you ever sit down to enjoy a good meal and come away feeling that it wasn't worth the trouble? The first few mouthfuls are pleasant, but after that the mechanical routine of shoving the food in begins and by the end of the meal you feel overfull and uncomfortable. The next thing most people do is to reach for some antacid in an effort to reduce discomfort. The antacid mixes with stomach acid and inactivates it. This may remove the symptoms but it does not remove the underlying causes, which are faulty habits and mental tension acting through the autonomic nervous system. For this, a system such as yoga is required.

When people talk about 'indigestion' they are really talking about dyspepsia, one of the most common ailments afflicting our present day civilization. It is a condition of the stomach in which digestive juices are incorrectly secreted and discomfort results.

The following symptoms are common in dyspepsia:

1. *Abdominal pain* with a burning sensation may be present. This should be differentiated by an experienced doctor from ulcer pain which is gnawing in nature. Usually there is a feeling of fullness or bloating, which may range from mild to severe.

2. *Heartburn* is the result of acid reflux from the stomach and produces burning behind the breastbone, just in front of the heart. Because of this it must be differentiated

from potentially serious heart disease such as angina pectoris and other chest diseases which have similar symptoms. Heartburn is caused by movement of gastric juices out of the stomach and into the oesophagus so that the burning travels upwards.

3. *Belching* can occur because of anxiety, wind producing foods, or obstruction to the outlet of the stomach (which leads to stagnation). Wind can be passed out either through the mouth or anus. Belching may also be self-induced in an effort to relieve the persisting discomfort.

4. *Regurgitation* of gastric contents occurs with a combination of belching and acid reflux, especially after a very large meal. Air, food and acids travel up into the throat or into the mouth where they leave a very bitter taste.

Because most people are not aware of the potential of yoga to eliminate indigestion problems, a few attacks of dyspepsia take them to visit their doctor where they seek both medication and psychological support. A typical conversation goes like this:

• When does this burning feeling start?
• As soon as I get up in the morning, doctor.
• How long does it last?
• For a good part of the day, though it's not as bad in the evening. It is worse when I feel nervous or when I have eaten too much or too quickly.

From this sort of interview the doctor will try to find out what is the underlying problem causing the discomfort. It is important that people suffering from indigestion visit a doctor so as to eliminate the possibility of more serious diseases. Then they can start to remove the underlying causes which can be simply summed up as 'too much, too fast, too rich and too tense'.

Overindulgence

Eating too much is the first cause of dyspepsia. At the physical level this is generally a case of one's eyes being bigger than one's stomach. When we have the choice of

93

endless assortments of delicious foods, how many of us have the willpower and common sense to eat sensibly? In most cases we become a slave to the passions of our taste and overindulge by trying this or that, and "just a little bit more, thanks, even though I'm really quite full". Indeed many hosts and hostesses are offended if you do not show your approval of their hospitality by eating and drinking as much as you can. Under these circumstances it is amazing how much some people can pack away.

Eating too much often leads to eating too quickly, the next phase in the cause of dyspepsia. If we want to eat a large quantity of food, it stands to reason that we will have to eat it more quickly. This has a twofold purpose. Firstly, it allows us to eat more in the same time as it would take to eat a normal meal and secondly, it looks like "we really didn't eat so much".

Eating too much too quickly prevents us from really enjoying and savouring the food. It also prevents adequate mastication, which sets the digestive process off to a bad start. Saliva is not mixed properly, nor is the food completely broken down. Large particles travel into the stomach and require extra energy to digest. The correct quantities of alkaline saliva, acidic gastric juice and enzymes are not secreted and indigestion results.

Many people eat too quickly because they are not relaxed and centred in the present. They are anxious, worried about some past action or future event, and find it difficult to be aware of eating and to enjoy their food. Others get caught up in the anticipation of the next pleasure and start looking forward to more food even before finishing the first round.

Rich and spicy foods may also cause dyspepsia or aggravate an already existing condition, as do chocolate, coffee and acidic fruit juices. Smoking and drinking alcohol just before eating are also implicated. Usually however, tasty foods cause indigestion through the fact that we tend to eat more than our capacity.

Delving deeper

There are three important facets of dyspepsia which lie under the surface manifestations of discomfort and heartburn. They are related to tension in (i) swadhisthana chakra, (ii) manipura chakra, (iii) the environment, usually as a by-product of tension in these two chakras.

Swadhisthana chakra is related to pleasure and preservation of the species. The two main mechanisms used to satisfy its innate urges are sex and food. If there is any discord in the sexual aspects of our lives and we are not deriving enough satisfaction and fulfilment, we tend to sublimate by overeating. According to yogic physiology, taste is the sensation that is associated with swadhisthana chakra.

Tension in manipura chakra can occur when energy from a blockage in swadhisthana spills over. If we cannot satisfy our sexual urge and if at the same time we are suffering from dyspepsia because of overeating, then all avenues to swadhisthana are blocked and frustration occurs. At the same time, these frustrations spill over into the environment causing problems with family, work and so on. This results in rage and anger or in depression, which are tensions in manipura chakra.

Problems with the external environment such as quarrels in the family or with friends, troubles at work, threatened dismissal from a job or even promotion with added responsibilities, cause tension and overstimulate the sympathetic nervous system. Any physical, emotional or mental pain stimulates the sympathetic system, thereby stopping the movements of the stomach and slowing down the secretion of digestive juices. This means that any food eaten at such times remains in the stomach longer. It is not digested properly and the nutrients cannot be fully absorbed. Furthermore, eating under continual emotional and mental tension is not pleasurable.

In experiments on dogs provoked into rage, little or no gastric secretion could be evoked, to the extent that even after the dogs had calmed down, a subsequent feeding, which usually acts as a very strong stimulus, had no effect. In this context H.W. Davenport says: "Similar suppression of secretion in rage has been found in man, and literature from the most ancient times contains anecdotes describing cessation of digestion during episodes of sympathetic discharge."[1]

Overcoming the causative factors

Some people use bicarbonate of soda to relieve their dyspepsia but this is not recommended by medical authorities because the gas it produces distends the stomach and may perforate an ulcer if there is already one there. Other antacids such as magnesium trisilicate and aluminium hydroxide are preferred. Doctors will combine these with sedatives or tranquillizers if there is an obvious emotional component and will give some dietary instructions to eliminate the causative food factors. Rarely, however, do people try to reduce their emotional and psychological problems. This is because they view dyspepsia as a physical disorder and so they seek a physical cure or means of relief. Yoga therapy stresses the mental and emotional factors as fundamental components of cure and this is the basis of its success, for in this way it eliminates stress.

Each person handles stress in their own way. Some people become upset while others take it in their stride. Those people who are easily distressed get dyspepsia. For them, yoga is the best way to deal with their problems for it quickly eliminates tension and gradually strengthens the body and mind so that they are not so easily affected by stressful situations. As the health improves so does the ability so solve those problems which were once the root cause of dyspepsia.

We need to find a way to tame the animal within us, which comes in the form of the autonomic nervous system. This system goes on by itself without the need for conscious direction by the will and it reacts blindly to both joy and rage. Yoga teaches us to become aware of and then to control its function by developing the attitude of a detached witness. Experiments with biofeedback have proven this fact to the scientific world. Yoga has also been proven to consciously control the autonomic system and prevent the emotional highs and lows from affecting our bodies.

Yoga helps us to relax so that we can eat slowly with enjoyment. By developing awareness we become sensitive to our body's needs rather than to its desires and can then stop eating when we have had enough. Eventually the practices create a desire for more pure and simple foods which make us feel better. As we learn to balance our inner energies we find that we need to eat less. When yogic awareness is slowly and carefully cultivated, most diseases, especially self-induced ones such as dyspepsia, drop away automatically without effort on our part. This is true relaxation.

Dyspepsia sadhana

The following practices will eliminate tension, which is the root cause of dyspepsia, and help to restore the digestive system to normal functioning. Choose those which suit you best:

- *Hatha yoga shatkriya*: Kunjal and neti, vyaghra kriya, agnisar kriya, nauli, vastra dhauti, shankhaprakshalana (to be practised only under expert guidance).
  Note: These shatkriyas are not to be practised if an ulcer is present.
- *Asana*: Pawanmuktasana parts 1 and 2, vajrasana, shashankasana, bhujangasana, shavasana.
- *Pranayama*: Bhramari, seetkari, nadi shodhana.
- *Meditation*: Yoga nidra, antar mouna, chidakasha dharana. These practices, though sufficient in themselves, can be combined with karma yoga, bhakti yoga and jnana yoga for faster, deeper and more long-term results.

97

13

Wind

Everyone has wind, also called flatus or flatulence. It is a completely natural process for the body to produce gases from its myriad chemical reactions in the digestive system. There comes a point, though, when excessive wind becomes a problem, causing us or others discomfort. One becomes aware of passing more wind than usual, perhaps accompanied by pain or an offensive odour.

Gas formation

Under normal circumstances a certain amount of air is swallowed with food, drink and saliva. Some gas is belched while the remainder passes into the intestines. Of this, some is absorbed, but most, particularly the nitrogen, is expelled from the rectum. Some gases such as carbon dioxide are produced in the intestine. Carbohydrate digestion and the interaction of alkaline pancreatic secretions and acid stomach juices form approximately three to four litres per day, most of which is absorbed. Hydrogen sulphide, which gives the contents of the bowel its peculiar and occasionally offensive smell, can form from proteins, legumes (peas, beans and dal), cauliflower, cabbage, and brussel sprouts.

The major gas areas shown on X-ray are the stomach and the colon. Very little is seen in the small intestine. In the normal situation, pressure in the stomach is greater than pressure in the chest, so that one would expect any gas to be forced out of the stomach in the form of belching. This is prevented, however, by a sphincter or valve between the stomach and the oesophagus that can withstand this pressure. The stomach can accept a large volume of food without an appreciable rise in pressure, but a heavy meal, with large amounts of swallowed gas or carbon dioxide generated by the combination of bicarbonate and gastric acid, increases the pressure. Then at the next swallow, when the sphincter relaxes, belching occurs and the gastric contents may be forced upwards.

The gas in the colon is formed from the action of bacteria dissolving the walls of intact fruit and vegetable particles, which are composed of cellulose. These particles should have been broken down in cooking or by the teeth so that their contents were released and made available for absorption into the bloodstream from the small intestine.

People with bad food habits, who are tense and rush through their meals, do not break down the cell walls properly as they do not give sufficient time to chewing. As there is no way to digest cellulose above the colon, intact particles move through the intestines until they reach the colon where bacteria with the capacity to digest cellulose are present. These liberate the cell contents which ferment, releasing gas.

Probably the most common cause of excessive gas is the swallowing of air, which may be due to anxiety or the abdominal discomfort of dyspepsia, peptic ulcer or any other process which induces waterbrash and the excessive swallowing of saliva and air. For example, many people feel full after eating only a small amount of food and may assume this is due to wind. In actual fact, however, most cases are due to dyspepsia. In an attempt to relieve discomfort and release wind, many people take in a little air and then regurgitate it. This becomes a habit although it brings little relief and these people still complain of bloating, distension, belching and so on. Some gas is belched and the rest passes out of the stomach and down into the intestines.

Taming the wind

Removing wind problems is really quite easy if we follow the recommended program along with the observance of a few simple, sensible suggestions.

1. Become aware that you are swallowing air and regurgitating it, and then start to remedy the real cause of your discomfort, which is dyspepsia.
2. Chew your food well. The amount of chewing required will vary according to the texture of the food and also how well it is cooked.
3. Eat in relative silence. Some people talk during the meal more than they eat and subsequently they also take extra air in as they swallow.
4. Avoid excessive quantities of legumes, beans, lentils and other sulphur containing foods. The ideal ratio is one part legumes to four parts grain. In this way we gain the optimal amount of protein with the least amount of sulphur released, so that less hydrogen sulphide is formed.

Wind sadhana

The following practices will greatly alleviate wind problems. Select those which suit you best.

- *Hatha yoga shatkriya*: Kunjal and neti, vyaghra kriya, basti, shankhaprakshalana (under guidance) and laghoo shankhaprakshalana.
- *Asana*: Pawanmuktasana part 2, surya namaskara, vajrasana (especially after meals), shashankasana, ardha matsyendrasana, bhujangasana, paschimottanasana.
- *Pranayama*: Nadi shodhana, bhramari, ujjayi.
- *Meditation*: Yoga nidra.

14

What's Eating You?

It is a recognized fact in both the yogic tradition and in medical science that peptic ulcers have their roots in the mind and are partly a direct consequence of mental tension and worry. In this stress filled day and age it is estimated that at least one person in ten is likely to have a peptic ulcer at one time or another.

Ulcers form by the action of bacteria called Helicobacter Pyloris which, under the right conditions, are able to attack and infect the lining of the stomach and upper small intestine. This allows the gastric juices to burn a hole in the stomach lining, causing either a discreet ulcer or multiple, pinpoint bleeding spots called gastritis. The ulcer is a crater, a raw and bleeding depression in the stomach lining, similar in appearance to those on the moon.

There are two main types of peptic ulceration:
1. *Gastric ulcers* which occur inside the stomach.
2. *Duodenal ulcers* which occur near the junction of the duodenum and the stomach.

The cause of ulcers

A mind filled with tension and worry, unexpressed and blocked emotions, stressful situations, personality problems, poor lifestyle and genetic predisposition are thought to be major factors in causing ulcers. Smoking, alcohol and dietary indiscretions are secondary factors aggravating the underlying condition. In India excessive consumption of chillies, spicy foods, which are irritants of the gastric lining, and mental tension lead to chronic peptic ulcer and also further aggravate the condition when the ulcer has developed.

Ulcer patients are often highly-strung, excitable and ambitious people who are leading very active lives. Society sets high goals which these people feel they have to attain to be successful in their own eyes and in the eyes of others. Most ulcer sufferers are attempting many things at once and worry about the results of their undertakings. These are the people who cannot rest, even when the have the chance. They may sleep too little and take insufficient food or alternatively smoke, drink and eat excessively because of underlying mental tension.

Many ulcer patients fall into a distinct personality group. They are usually the type of people who handle their emotional drives internally, tending to 'bottle up' their worries and problems. That is, instead of becoming angry and relieving their tension or creatively channelling excess emotional energy externally, they internalize it. Perhaps this is because they are afraid to let people see how they feel, so they channel this energy into their nervous systems and internal organs. Then, if their body has its predisposed weak point in the stomach, ulcers can develop. This type of person allows worries and problems to gain the upper hand so that emotional energy literally eats them! With these people it is not a question of what they eat, so much as 'what is eating them'. The negative energy at the mental, emotional level is transmitted into the body as a negative, self-destructive energy which eats into the lining of the stomach as well as their emotional and mental well-being.

The effects of anger and the emotions have been researched using hypnotism. Hypnotized subjects were placed in front of an X-ray machine and the suggestion was made that they feel anger. X-rays showed the stomach tense up, constrict and then go into spasm, indicating that it was grossly affected by tension.

Other experiments have shown that depression or fear tend to slow down gastric acid production while anger, resentment and hostility increase it. Emotional imbalance triggers the limbic system of the brain to readjust the nervous-endocrine system via the hypothalamus, which affects both the autonomic system and the endocrine glands. If this emotional imbalance is inappropriate and ongoing rather than short-term and justified, then the whole delicate balance between acid secretion and the production of protective mucus is upset. According to yogic theory this sets up the correct conditions for bacteria to grow, affecting the lining of the stomach and allowing the acid to eat into the muscle coating.

Other factors thought to be involved in the formation of ulcers are certain drugs such as aspirin. Seasonal factors can also play a part; for example, in Britain there is an increased death rate from ulcers during winter.

Peptic ulcers tend to run in families. The children of parents with duodenal ulcers tend to get duodenal ulcers. This is especially true when ulcers occur in childhood or adolescence. Though it used to be thought that this indicated that ulcers were caused by a genetic weakness, more recent research shows that the early environment we grow up in plays an important role. Not only do children inherit physical characteristics and weaknesses, but they also develop some of the same personality traits as their parents, the same tendencies that caused them to develop ulceration.

The social and economic environment is also important as gastric ulcers tend to be more common amongst the poor, while duodenal ulcers are evenly distributed throughout the population.

An interesting relationship between sex and ulcer exists. Duodenal ulcers occur five to ten times more commonly in men than women, while rupture of the ulcer (a serious complication) occurs 20 times more often in men. This is probably due in most part to the differences in life pattern of men and women. However, it is thought that the female sex hormones play a significant part in protecting women. During pregnancy, for example, active, acute ulcers are virtually unknown and the symptoms which cease soon after pregnancy begin to recommence after delivery.

Whatever the contributing causes to the occurrence of peptic ulcers, it seems that the major problem is mental tension interfering with the balance of stomach acid versus stomach mucosal resistance.

Do you have an ulcer?

The three most important symptoms of ulcer are chronic dyspepsia (discomfort after meals), pain and bleeding. Ulcer sufferers quite often have episodes of dyspepsia for many months before discovering they have an ulcer. This, or pain, usually takes them to the doctor. The pain is generally described as a gnawing or burning sensation found in the upper abdomen, just under the sternum of the rib cage, in the midline or just slightly to the right.

Duodenal ulcer pain tends to occur between meals and is characteristically relieved by food, especially milk. It is described as 'hunger pain' and may awaken the sufferer from sleep between 2 and 4 a.m. Gastric ulcer pain occurs mainly one hour after eating, is not relieved by taking food and only rarely occurs at night.

In both cases the pain is episodic, that is, it occurs daily for days or weeks at a time and then disappears, only to reappear weeks or months later. Between attacks the individual feels perfectly healthy and can eat and drink without apparent harm. However, with time the episodes of pain become longer and the period between the episodes diminishes. This is especially so when dietary indiscretions or alcoholic excesses frequently occur.

Other symptoms are feelings of discomfort and distension, loss of appetite, nausea, vomiting and weight loss (especially in gastric ulcers). Heartburn (bringing up of gastric contents into the throat or mouth) and waterbrash (excessive salivation caused by nausea) can also occur.

Bleeding from an acute ulcer can lead to vomiting bright red blood from the mouth and black blood appearing in the faeces. It may also appear as anaemia or even cause acute shock from sudden loss of blood.

The psychosomatics of ulcers

The ulcer personality tends to be dynamic and fiery and is prone to the suppression of jealousy and anger. Thus the energy travels into the stomach where it causes excessive acid secretion and makes one more susceptible to ulcers.

Wolf and Wolff studied the case of a man whose stomach had been perforated by a bullet.[1] The wound did not heal completely but formed a fistula, a passage through the stomach and abdominal walls by which the interior of the stomach could be seen. During depression, gastric secretion was reduced and it was subnormal for several months when the dominant psychic state was self-reproach. When the same subject was unjustly reproached, he experienced strong feelings of hostility and the blood supply and subsequent acid secretion increased by about 25%, remaining elevated for two weeks. The mucosa (lining) became engorged, wet, swollen and dark – that is, full of blood. The general conclusion was that emotional states such as fear, sadness or withdrawal appear to reduce gastric secretion, whereas aggressiveness or the will to fight back appear to increase it.

Another experiment involved pairs of monkeys who were restrained and subjected to electric shocks delivered to the feet automatically every 20 seconds for six hours. After a six hour rest, shocks were again repeated for 6 hours, and so on. The first monkey, the 'executive', was given a lever to press. When pressed at the right time, it prevented shocks to both monkeys and he quickly learned to stop the shocks. His partner, the 'control', received very few shocks. His lever was without effect and so he soon came to ignore it. The executive monkeys died after several days of continuous stress from gastrointestinal erosion and bleeding. No control monkey died or had ulceration.

People with ulcers tend to be like monkey number one, the 'executive', except that they are not forced into their situation by anyone other than themselves. These people are power dominant personalities who want to prove themselves to themselves and to their peer group. They feel insecure when they are not in a position of power, and because no one can achieve total power they are never without some insecurity and tension, even in their dealings with themselves. They can sometimes be seen on their holidays walking by the sea, directing the action of the waves. This personality reflects tension in the manipura chakra area and therefore sadhana is directed towards its relaxation.

Treatment

Medical science prescribes a course of very strong antibiotics, which have proved a boon in treating acute ulcers. It is a personal decision whether one wants to use antibiotics alone, or a combination of both. It is best to discuss your options with your therapist.

From the yogic point of view, rest and relaxation are acknowledged as being major factors in relieving serious, acute and chronic ulcer problems. In the field of rest and relaxation yoga is unsurpassed. All yoga practices, whether asana or meditation techniques, are intended to remove tension in all its forms, whether physical, emotional or mental. These practices allow the nervous system and consequently the digestive system to return to normal. This applies to all digestive problems, not just ulcers.

Furthermore, yoga creates a deeper understanding and tolerance of both oneself and others. This encourages each of us to live a more harmonious and happy life. Developing such feelings as optimism and confidence gives us a higher level of resistance to ward off diseases and problems and allows the body to better heal itself. Therefore, we can say that yoga is the way to remove not only the symptoms but also the root cause – mental tension and poor lifestyle.

Yogic therapy should be used in conjunction with medical treatment for the best combination of methods to alleviate both the pain, distress and underlying tensions. Apart from any medication, the acute ulcer is treated with rest. Milk diet eases pain and antacids help to relieve excessive acid. At best this symptomatic form of treatment is only good for a short while until yogic relaxation practices have rebalanced the mind and nervous system so that the root cause is removed.

Medical management of ulcer symptoms, though effective, may not prevent the ulcer from recurring, nor will it prevent the natural tendency of ulcer symptoms to increase and decrease.

A liquid or light, bland diet is to be taken until the ulcer heals completely. Only then should the normal diet be resumed. This bland diet should be taken every two or three hours and each meal should be small. These small regular meals throughout the day will help to protect the ulcer crater from the acids and give it a chance to heal. Rough foods such as bran, coarse cereals, leafy vegetables, grated carrots, etc, should be avoided along with all oily and spicy foods like chilli, pepper, rich sauces, curries, salad dressings, mustard, cheese, nuts, chutneys, fried food, cakes, etc. The following diet is recommended:

1. Bread, chapatti, toast, crackers
2. Finely ground, well cooked cereals such as cream of wheat, cream of rice, semolina, barley, etc.
3. Milk, cream, buttermilk, cottage cheese, cream cheese, cream soups
4. Apple sauce, ripe bananas, pears, prunes, apricots (all without skins), fruit juices, citrus juice diluted with water
5. Vegetables such as carrots, squash, peas, asparagus, mashed or baked potatoes (without the skin) can be cooked in a little water but not fried
6. Macaroni, noodles, spaghetti, butter, margarine, olive oil
7. Poached or scrambled eggs; for meat-eaters only broiled lamb or chicken.

This diet is designed to provide essential food materials in an easily digestible form and is valuable for ulcers, colitis and other intestinal complaints. We do not, however, recommend this diet for general use; it should only be followed until the ulcer has healed.

Eventually a normal diet can be resumed, but it will always be necessary, even after the ulcer has completely healed, to be very careful about the following:

- Fried food
- Pickles, curries, chilli, pepper, ginger, mustard
- Tobacco and alcohol in any form
- Excess tea or coffee, especially strong and black

Rest is essential in healing an ulcer, and until it has healed complete rest is suggested. As strength is regained it is possible to commence yogic techniques which, when practised under expert guidance, are designed to reduce mental tension, give control over the autonomic nervous system and thus prevent a recurrence.

Ulcer sadhana

Until the ulcer has completely healed, the only practices that should be performed are as follows:

- *Hatha yoga shatkriya*: Neti.
- *Asana*: Pawanmuktasana part 1, shavasana, vajrasana, shashankasana.
- *Pranayama*: Nadi shodhana, bhramari, seetkari, ujjayi.
- *Meditation*: Yoga nidra, antar mouna.

Later, when healing of the acute ulcer is complete, kunjal kriya can be added to the cleansing techniques. A yoga ashram is an excellent place to recuperate after an acute attack because it provides a positive atmosphere away from worries and tensions.

15

Feeling Constipated?

Constipation is a common complaint which people every-where, from all age groups suffer from at one time or another. Constipation should be taken as a warning sign, even though in itself it is a simple and easily curable con-dition. If you do not correct the condition when it arises, then you may be allowing the process which causes con-stipation to snowball into more serious diseases such as arthritis and perhaps even lethal diseases such a arterio-sclerosis and colonic cancer. The amazing thing that most people will appreciate is that it can be so easily remedied by the regular practice of yogic techniques.

Constipation means the infrequent or difficult passage of hard, dry faeces. It is not just the irregularity of the stools, but the hardness and dryness of the faeces that makes it so difficult and produces dissatisfaction with bowel activity. The major symptoms, apart from difficulty in passing stool, are headache, malaise, gas, loss of appetite, possibly nausea, foul smelling breath, a furred tongue, heaviness and dis-comfort in the abdomen.

CONSTIPATION IN PERSPECTIVE

What is a normal stool?
The average person passes one large, well formed stool per day. However, some people enjoy good health and pass only

two or three stools per week. Thus, every individual must assess for themselves what their 'normal' is, and not try to compare themselves with other people. In Britain, fewer than 10% of the people have less than one motion per day and only 1% have a motion less frequently than three times a week. In Britain, these latter are classed as constipated. However, hard and difficult to pass stools indicate constipation no matter what the frequency of motion. On a typical low residue diet, people in western countries rarely have more than three motions per day, whereas the high residue diet of other countries makes three motions per day normal.

Are irregular motions unhealthy?

Many people believe that they must pass a good motion every day, regularly like clockwork. Of course, this is a good habit to get into but it is not essential for good health. Often this belief can lead to neurosis and create more problems than it is worth, especially if we fail to live up to our expectations and beliefs. Some people actually suffer from imaginary constipation wherein the stools appear normal by ordinary standards but do not measure up to their expectations. These people attribute their neurotic symptoms such as exhaustion, lack of energy, back pain, memory loss, insomnia and loss of appetite to impaired elimination. When they develop neurosis they can then progress to real, and not just imagined, constipation caused by straining, mental tension and disharmony in the whole body. Try to develop regularity but do not worry if you do not stick to a rigid timetable of defecation. Much depends on regularity of diet, type of food consumed, the season and psychological health. But please remember...

Constipation is not fatal in itself!

To prove this, there was a case recorded by Geib and Jones where a man did not go to the toilet for one year from June 18, 1900 to June 21, 1901.[1] Before the faeces were removed, he belched a good deal and suffered some pain, had a distended abdomen, felt weak and lost some weight. However, after the removal of a mass of faeces weighing 100 pounds, he recovered rapidly. This case is obviously an extreme one, but it illustrates the fact that we will not die from constipation, although the clogging of our eliminative channels will ultimately lead to bad health, loss of energy and perhaps even serious disease.

Can constipation cause auto-intoxication?

The answer is not a simple, clear cut yes or no. There is no way for faeces, metabolized poisons or other toxins to be reabsorbed back into the body through the mucus membranes once they are expelled. Only water and salts are reabsorbed. However, we do feel unwell when we are constipated. This may be caused by a clogging of the eliminative system at a physical and pranic level, preventing toxins from coming out.

It is still uncertain why the symptoms of constipation occur. Auto-intoxication was a popular theory which, with little evidence for support, was discarded by most scientists and doctors. Experiments point to the fact that symptoms of constipation are mechanical in origin, that is they are caused by the stretching of tissues. *Samson Wright's Applied Physiology* demonstrates this point adequately.[2] Healthy men, who normally emptied their bowels only once or twice daily, withheld defecation for four days during which time they developed all the symptoms of supposed auto-intoxication such as foul breath, a furred tongue, impaired appetite, flatulence, nausea, lowered attention span, depression, restlessness, headache, insomnia and irritability. X-rays taken with a special contrast medium (a barium meal) showed all the food was in the colon while the small intestine was empty. When an enema was administered and the bowel evacuated, distress was alleviated. The subjects felt normal after one to two hours. If auto-intoxication had actually occurred, relief would have been much longer in coming.

111

These results were duplicated by packing masses of cotton wool or by inflating a balloon inside the rectum.

Auto-intoxication seems to be an imaginary condition which is made worse by fear of its consequences. The consequences, in the form of tension, heaviness, loss of energy, headache, laxative abuse, and subsequent deterioration of the zest for life, are very real however.

Are laxatives a good means to overcome this problem?

The answer to this is a definite 'No!' Laxatives can only cause more harm than good in the long term. Many people use them habitually because they fear constipation. When they try to stop using them, however, they have more trouble defecating because the laxatives have (i) cleaned out the whole digestive tract so that there is nothing left to defecate, and (ii) weakened the muscles of the intestines. This can lead to further fear of constipation and thus to the use of laxatives again. This vicious circle can easily be broken, however, with the help of yoga.

Cause of constipation

Constipation is a signal that all is not well within. Something is beginning to malfunction and should be corrected before worse damage occurs. The mechanism of metabolism functions on an input/output basis. That is, we put food into our bodies (whether in the form of solid, liquid or gas) and we expel wastes that are unwanted (such as faeces, urine and carbon dioxide). Thus the body is in balance. However, if our balance is upset for some reason or other, we can either find ourselves putting out too much or too little, and this will affect our input.

In constipation we are not eliminating waste efficiently. The body systems are upset. When the faeces are hard and dry, it means that there may be imbalance in secretion of juices from the stomach, intestines, liver, pancreas or other glands, or perhaps the absorption of water and salts is excessive. The point to remember is that there is imbalance and this is what must be corrected. There are two types of constipation:

1. **Colic constipation** occurs when there is a delay in movement of faeces into the rectum but the act of defecation is normal. This may be caused by a diet containing very little roughage, fibre or residue. Without the stimulus from roughage, the muscles become lazy and do not effectively push the faeces along. Other intestinal ailments, pain and the presence of fecaliths (masses of hard, dry faeces which obstruct or slow down peristalsis) can cause constipation by curtailing normal muscular movements.

2. **Dyschezic constipation** is a condition in which the faeces arrive normally at the pelvic colon, but their final evacuation is not adequately performed. If defecation is neglected, the wall relaxes and the desire passes away. In time, excessive distension occurs and the ability of the walls to contract, even with effort, becomes impaired. Small amounts of faeces are passed but the majority remains and distension continues.

One of the most important factors involved here is the habitual tendency to ignore the natural urge to go to the toilet, which interferes with the nervous system and its defecation reflex. An obstruction in the region of the rectum, taking the form of a polyp (a small outgrowth of mucosa), a foreign body (any object placed inside), or a tumour, can interfere with defecation. Some amazing foreign body obstructions, for example, a 40 watt electric light bulb and a tool case complete with tools, have been removed from the rectum and sigmoid colon.[3] However, this must be the least common cause of constipation.

Other factors involved in the dyschezic type are:

Mental tension: If we are tense or we strain when going to the toilet, our sympathetic nervous system is activated. This results in the opposite effect to that desired: the sphincters of the intestines close and the bowel wall expands to hold more faeces. In order to defecate properly, we should stimulate our parasympathetic nervous system by relaxing our minds and bodies. This contracts the bowel walls and pushes the faeces forward. There is no need to exert effort when you go to the toilet or to fear constipation. Fear only makes the condition worse. Defecation is automatic, like breathing. All we have to do is relax and be aware of the process. Trying too hard only causes further problems such as hernia, piles, prolapse and ulceration. In the elderly, straining may cause fainting or even death from a fatal cardiovascular accident.

Lack of energy: When we have mental problems such as depression, anxiety and other neuroses, we have to expend energy to maintain these states of mind, as they are unnatural and forced. They deplete our energy level and the physical body finds itself without sufficient energy to function efficiently. Thus the glands do not secrete, or when they do they secrete asynchronously so that their work is ineffective. At the same time, the muscles do not have sufficient force to propel the intestinal contents.

Another factor that reduces energy and makes it difficult to defecate is bad toilet training and the anxiety of trying to defecate without success. Bad training is probably at the root of all our problems and is the reason why we have to relearn to perform these simple body functions properly at later stages in our lives. It is for this reason that yoga is so valuable, re-educating us in how to live correctly and with a healthy frame of mind.

Fats slow down the propulsion of faeces and therefore should be reduced or eliminated from the diet. Meat and other low fibre foods such as refined flour, carbohydrate and fatty foods do not travel quickly through the intestine and as a result lead to constipation. This low fibre diet has also been linked with haemorrhoids, which are caused by straining at stool, and colonic (large intestinal) cancer. This is opposed to the high fibre content diet consisting of grains (whole and unrefined), fruits, vegetables and pulses, which helps to relieve both constipation and haemorrhoids. A copious supply of water should be maintained so as to keep the body well hydrated and to allow plenty of water to remain inside the intestines as lubrication for the faeces.

Psychology of constipation

Constipation can only occur in the body if there is constipation in the mind. Generally, people who are constipated do not like to give out. They are tight and hold their feelings in. Constipation is associated with mooladhara chakra which governs the possessions, security and self-preservation aspects of the personality. The tendency towards tightness and holding in is therefore concerned with insecurity which leads to the hoarding of material possessions or perhaps to a deeper disharmony in the relationship between the individual and their environment.

Perhaps there is also a deep-seated, subconscious fear of letting go and enjoying oneself. This may be further compounded by excessive toilet training coupled with the fear of being constipated. Not only are some people unable to defecate easily and naturally, but they fear that if they miss going to the toilet for even one day, serious complications will result.

Fortunately, yogic sadhana makes it very easy to overcome such problems. The appropriate practices relax tension associated with the mooladhara chakra and this automatically relieves the situation.

Suggestions for removing constipation

1. *Visit your doctor* for a thorough medical examination to ensure that there is no serious underlying cause for your constipation. When you know that there is nothing seriously wrong, you feel more relaxed.
2. *Do not listen* to many expert opinions. One is usually more than enough. Some people may make you worry unnecessarily, causing more constipation in the process.
3. *Exercise regularly.* This is one of the best preventions for constipation. Inactivity depletes the body of energy, allowing it to degenerate. City life with all the modern

115

conveniences at hand can induce laziness and the build-up of toxins within the body. Yoga exercises help to relax and empty out the bowels. For city dwellers and sedentary workers with reduced access to physical work, asanas and pranayama are the ideal replacement.

4. *Regulate* the volume of stool and the frequency of defecation by adding cereal bran (chilka) and plenty of fruit and vegetables to the diet. These foods contain cellulose, hemicellulose and lignin, which add bulk and thereby stimulate intestinal movement. Furthermore, cellulose and hemicellulose are partly digested by bacteria in the colon with the formation of fatty acids. These act as natural laxatives.

5. *Drink plenty of liquids.* Upon arising drink two glasses of warm water with lemon and a pinch of salt if you are not practising laghoo shankhaprakshalana.

6. *Reduce your dependence* on commercial laxatives as much as possible. If you are on purgatives and don't want to give them up straight away, we suggest that you change to a mild detergent-based laxative and then give this up also after a month of gradual withdrawal.

7. *Try to establish* a regular bowel habit at a suitable time during the day, especially in the morning before breakfast as this is the time when you are most likely to be relaxed – mentally, emotionally and physically. Do not worry if you do not achieve this immediately and do not strain.

8. *Remove chronic tension* which plays a vital role in constipation. One of the basic aims of yoga is to bring mental and emotional peace into one's life. As such, all yogic practices have an indirect contribution to make in removing constipation. Most commercial cures aim at removing the symptoms, namely the physical constipation. Yoga, on the other hand, aims at the root cause – mental and emotional constipation. If this more subtle form of constipation is removed, then the physical by-products will also disappear in just a short time.

Constipation sadhana

The yogic method par excellence for removing constipation is laghoo shankhaprakshalana. In this technique, saline water and certain asanas are used to clean the whole gastrointestinal tract. This is one of the most direct, dynamic and effective methods of removing constipation. It is simple to perform and takes only half an hour in the morning. No other technique is necessary for immediate relief; however, to tone up the rest of the body and remove constipation completely the use of other practices is recommended. Laghoo shankhaprakshalana can lead up to or follow on from a full course of shankhaprakshalana, but this requires expert guidance for its successful practice.

To overcome problems associated with mooladhara chakra practise pawanmuktasana part 2, moola bandha and ashwini mudra. These are of particular benefit in relaxing the deeper tensions related to this area of the personality.

The following practices generally help to alleviate constipation and its underlying causes. Select those that suit you best:

• *Hatha yoga shatkriya*: Agnisar and nauli kriyas, moola shodhana, basti.
• *Asana*: Surya namaskara, paschimottanasana, bhujang-asana, shalabhasana, dhanurasana, sarvangasana, ardha matsyendrasana.
• *Pranayama*: Nadi shodhana, bhastrika, ujjayi.
• *Meditation*: Yoga nidra, antar mouna, chidakasha dharana.

16

Painful Piles

Haemorrhoids or piles, which commonly and usually occur with constipation, are caused by straining associated with the difficult passage of faeces. Despite popular opinion, they do not necessarily require surgical treatment and are potentially curable by simple yogic exercises. The same yogic techniques that remedy constipation can be used with amazing efficiency in haemorrhoids. If you treat one condition, you also treat the other.

Haemorrhoids are swellings of the veins around the outlet of the rectum. They appear as distended purple sacs, like varicose veins on the legs. Haemorrhoids are a common problem with all age groups and it is estimated that in the western hemisphere more than 50% of the population over 50 years of age have at least some haemorrhoidal formation, with or without any symptoms. Haemorrhoidal symptoms include: bright red blood, prolapse of the haemorrhoid, mucus discharge, anal irritation, itching, and anaemia (caused by blood loss). They are classified from mild to severe, depending on the degree of prolapse, that is, how much they protrude from the anus:

1. First degree haemorrhoids project into the anus.
2. Second degree are larger and prolapse on defecation, but come back into place spontaneously.
3. Third degree haemorrhoids prolapse at any time and must be pushed back manually.

Cause of haemorrhoids

Though haemorrhoids are associated with constipation and straining, they also occur in pregnancy, cirrhosis of the liver and as an inherited condition. As they may be found with cancer of the large bowel, a thorough medical check-up is recommended.

Mental tension is the primary cause of haemorrhoids. People who are always in a hurry often strain on the toilet because they want to finish quickly in order to do something else. These people live in the future and cannot enjoy the present. Instead of allowing defecation to be a relaxed and pleasurable experience, they rush through it and in the uncontrolled actions that follow, the tissues deform under the pressure of excessive tension and strain. Stress causes spasm of the anal muscle, although we may not be aware of it, and defecation is disturbed. The spasm increases the intra-rectal pressure leading to congestion of veins and straining; eventually haemorrhoids form.

When we are always straining downwards the body's energies adapt and form new patterns. The downward energies of apana (those involved in defecation, urination, the passing of flatus and the birth process) become predominant over the upward energies of prana (those involved in the breathing cycle) causing imbalance in the body. Unless we rectify this problem through yogic means, no cure can be permanent. This is why haemorrhoids reappear even after surgery, which is a painful and distressing procedure.

Diet is another factor implicated in the cause of haemorrhoids. Constipating, low fibre, high protein, high fat foods are hard to digest and transport through the intestines. Much energy is depleted in the effort to metabolize this diet. A sedentary lifestyle with little physical exercise further weakens the body and lowers the energies within. As a result, peristalsis, which requires an abundance of energy to work efficiently, is slowed down and there is not enough power left to make expulsion an enjoyable experience.

Reversing the condition

At the physical level we have to break down the tension that is causing the haemorrhoids to form. The first area to treat is tension in the haemorrhoidal area itself and the second is tension within the personality. Yoga offers the techniques to directly approach both these problems and to eliminate them.

Many doctors believe that haemorrhoids are a reversible condition and have based their procedures on this. Lord, who devised a relatively successful and widely used method, has based his procedure on the belief that "haemorrhoids constitute a reversible condition and that they are caused by a narrowing of the lower rectum and/or anal canal. The narrowing interferes with the normal processes of defecation and leads to an abnormal raising of the intrarectal pressure during the act, causing congestion and hence haemorrhoids."[1]

This raised pressure is a result of the increased energy in the lower abdomen from apana. Lord tried to disperse this tension by forcibly dilating the anus and thereby breaking the muscle spasm. Yoga uses a much more gentle approach, but with the same objective in mind. Moola shodhana massages and soothes swollen, inflamed haemorrhoidal tissue, and breaks up spasm. It also sends the stagnant, pooled energy and blood upward by stimulating the mooladhara chakra area. Only a few days of practice are necessary to give relief.

Modern medical therapy, on the other hand, offers the following treatment when piles are causing symptoms such as pain, itching, bleeding or discomfort.

1. *General measures* start with keeping the anal area clean and dry. This means that after every motion, the area should be washed with cold water and dried: toilet paper should be avoided. This is the traditional Indian method of hygiene and proves to be more soothing and sanitary (provided the hands are washed properly afterwards), because the cold water constricts the vascular tissue.

Regulation of bowel habit is another important item. For this a high fibre diet is recommended using bran, wholemeal bread or chappatis, fruits and vegetables, as well as plenty of fluids. This eliminates the constipation factor and may be all that is required for cure.

2. *Injection therapy* uses a corrosive substance which is injected into the haemorrhoid to create scar tissue. It is hoped that this will stop first degree haemorrhoids from developing into second and third degree, although this is unlikely unless the causative factors are removed.

3. *Rubber band ligation* is the tying of second and third degree internal haemorrhoids with an elastic band to strangle them and cause them to slough off. It has been quite successful and is painless. This method does not require hospitalization whereas an operation does.

4. *Operations* are of two types:
   i) Anal dilation such as Lord's procedure where eight fingers are inserted into the anus, which is subsequently stretched.
   ii) Excision of the haemorrhoid, an old, painful and time consuming procedure which is losing favour with many doctors. It should only be used when absolutely necessary and when other modes of treatment have failed. Surgery is unnecessary when one uses yogic techniques which remove the pain, bleeding and other symptoms of haemorrhoids, as well as the root cause.

Haemorrhoid sadhana

Haemorrhoids very rarely require urgent medical treatment, although occasionally they may bleed profusely and therefore it is worth your while to give some time to the following yogic techniques. These have been time tested and shown to remove the bodily and mental tension which causes spasm and constriction of the rectum muscles.

Haemorrhoid sadhana is divided into two main parts:
1. The alleviation of constipation (see chapter 15).

121

2. Specific practices for piles, which include the following:
   i) *Hatha yoga shatkriya*: Moola shodhana.
   ii) *Asana*: Sarvangasana or vipareeta karani asana (which drains stagnant blood from the anus).
   iii) *Mudra and bandha*: Ashwini mudra (can be practised on its own at any time of the day or with inverted asanas), moola bandha.

17

Diarrhoea

Diarrhoea, the antithesis of constipation, is a mysterious phenomenon in the minds of most people. When the urge to eliminate loose, watery stool becomes uncontrollable and very frequent, some people fear that, like a leaking vessel, they will soon be emptied of all their contents. However, in most cases, diarrhoea should not cause anxiety, for it can actually be a useful cleansing process if approached with the correct frame of mind. The increased frequency in diarrhoea is caused by increased peristaltic movement, which in turn may be due to either an increased volume of stool (perhaps because of excess water) or an increased tone in the colon wall (perhaps due to emotional excitement).

The question of what actually constitutes diarrhoea is a controversial subject. *Davidson's Principles and Practice of Medicine* says that "...less than 1% of the population (in Britain) have more than three bowel movements per day and this should be regarded as abnormal; particularly if the stool is not formed. When the stool is liquid, or semi-formed, it must be regarded as abnormal whatever the frequency of bowel movement. It should be realized that the diet in western countries is low in roughage whereas in countries where a high residue diet is usual, more than three bowel movements per day may be normal."[1]

In investigating diarrhoea, the doctor must determine whether the cause is mental, infective, allergic, due to

123

chemical poisoning, etc. To do this he will ask the following questions:
1. How many bowel movements are you having per day or night?
2. Is defecation difficult or painful?
3. What is the consistency of the stool?
4. Has there been any recent change of bowel habits?

It is important to differentiate, for example, functional (psychogenic) diarrhoea which tends to occur on rising in the morning, from infection or some organic disease in which diarrhoea usually occurs both during the day and at night.

The colon normally receives 400 to 500 millilitres of chyme (the substance in the small intestine which is the end product of digestion and assimilation). From this it produces about 150 grams of faeces per day, of which approximately 70% is water. In terms of water loss from the body, the faecal component plays a minor role in the normal situation.

In diarrhoea the water and electrolytes lost come from the small intestines. The intestines are normally presented with more than ten litres of liquid per day, which comes from diet and from secretions of the stomach, liver, pancreas and intestines. Of this only one hundredth remains unabsorbed in the faeces. Most is absorbed in the small intestine and only 300 to 400 millilitres in the large. In the case of diarrhoea, water is either not absorbed or is secreted in excess by the organs of the body. It is then sent along to the colon whose water holding capacity is very limited. Thus the urge to defecate comes quite often. In some cases this can be excessive, for example, in cholera where 75 litres of water may be lost in five days. This is because the cholera exotoxin causes the intestines to secrete copious fluid.

The urge to defecate is stimulated by the delivery of faeces to the rectum which becomes distended. In diarrhoea this fullness is not essential, the massive and strong contractions of a hyper-excitable colon are enough. If the contractions are strong enough, a sense of fullness of the rectum and a desire to defecate accompany each contraction despite emptiness of the rectum. If the contractions are very strong and repeated vigorously, the mucosa lining in the intestines may be rubbed off, causing bleeding.

Diarrhoea can be categorized as follows:

1. *Psychogenic*: psychological and not physical in origin.
2. *Acute*: major causes are infectious agents (viral, bacterial or parasitic), toxins, poisons and drugs.
3. *Chronic*: indicates underlying disease which can be found in almost any of the digestive organs from the stomach to the rectum, for example, oversecretion of gastric acid, cancer, ulcerative colitis, overactive thyroid, bacillary or amoebic dysentery, post-antibiotic therapy, etc.

NERVOUS DIARRHOEA

"Alterations in function of the colon frequently accompany emotional disturbances. The acute reaction to extreme fright is known to everyone and is described in familiar phrases of the common speech. Medical students facing a serious examination frequently have diarrhoea."[2]

No other organ system is as susceptible to psychological disturbances as the human gastrointestinal tract. Colonic neurosis is probably the truest example of a 'civilization' disorder. Most doctors will vouch for the fact that this common disorder, along with most of the other psycho-somatic digestive disorders, presents a long and often painful uphill battle that meets with little success and ultimately forces many sufferers to travel from one specialist to another in an attempt to find a cure. According to the findings of Cecil-Loeb: "This disorder is considered to account for more than 50% of all gastrointestinal illnesses and ranks with the common cold as one of the leading causes of recurrent minor disabilities."[3] A few lucky individuals come within the fold of yoga and find there the practical techniques necessary to eliminate the root cause.

Few physicians will doubt that the incidence of psycho-logically originated gastrointestinal disease will continue to increase under the pressures of modern living. In an effort to come to terms with this disorder and to increase understanding of it, various names have been given such as spastic colon (because the colon is in spasm and the muscles are stiff), mucus colitis (because mucus is sometimes found in the stool), nervous diarrhoea (because of its anxiety component), unstable colon, etc. Whatever its name however, it almost always results in discomfort and eventually a visit to the doctor.

The main symptoms are described as uncoordinated muscle action, abdominal pain, flatulence and either constipation or diarrhoea. Irregular movements of the colon and muscle spasm prevent faeces from moving properly and thus water may be reabsorbed during the time faeces are retained, causing constipation. Alternatively, it is shot out with considerable force at the most unexpected moments.

The irritable bowel syndrome

This syndrome is said to be more common in women than in men and usually occurs between the ages of 20 to 40 years. The condition occurs in highly emotional individuals and is characterized by loose stools on arising, after meals, and/or as a result of some situation producing emotional strain. The sufferer may become so conscious of, and so obsessed with, the condition that a visit to the theatre, travel, or any situation where there is no access to a toilet becomes impossible.

The commonest complaint in this condition is lower abdominal pain which occurs in attacks and is described as cramping and diffuse. It is relieved by defecation and may be provoked by eating, presumably because the nervous system is over-reactive due to mental and emotional strain. The individual complains of recurring attacks of abdominal pain lasting for some hours, but the pain is not very severe.

There are three main types of irritable bowel in which:
1. *Diarrhoea predominates* – this is a dysfunction of the motor (peristaltic) system which results in diarrhoea and painful

126

cramps. The motion itself, however, is painless and several loose, watery stools are passed per day, usually in the morning either before or after breakfast but hardly ever at night. It occurs intermittently; in mild cases the stool is normal between attacks. Diarrhoea may persist in the more severe cases, nearly crippling the lifestyle and forcing the sufferer to remain housebound.

2. *Constipation predominates* – this is mainly a dysfunction within the secretory system and its mucus production in which hard, pellet-like stools and mucus are passed.

3. *Diarrhoea and constipation alternate* – this is a dysfunction of both motor and secretory systems. During the periods of constipation many try to relieve the condition by taking laxatives which lead to another episode of diarrhoea and a vicious circle.

Other symptoms common to all three conditions are abdominal distension (especially after meals), intestinal rumbling and occasional nausea, loss of appetite and fatigue. There are no abdominal physical findings apart from fast pulse rate, brisk reflexes and so on, generally associated with a nervous and highly emotional personality.

The cause

This syndrome is one of mental diarrhoea, a functional, not an organic disorder. Though purely psychological in origin, it can manifest because the digestive system is weakened by unhealthy lifestyle, tension, fast pace of modern life, ambitions and interpersonal conflicts. Physical and mental fatigue also play an important role, as do the use of purgatives. The condition tends to occur in families, because children pick up many personality characteristics from their family.

Anything which causes fear or anger will affect this condition. Reactions to pain, fear and anxiety reduce the blood supply to the colon and, therefore, motility and the secretion of mucus. Anger, resentment and hostility, either overt or subconscious, increase the blood flow to the colon. This seems to be because each emotional reaction stimulates

127

a different chemical component of the sympathetic nervous system. According to Funkenstein, fear causes the body to secrete adrenaline while anger acts via noradrenaline.[4] Both substances act differently. Adrenaline causes the gut to relax and the sphincters to close. Noradrenaline is much less potent in this regard. Thus we see a difference in the effect of fear and anger.

In the irritable bowel syndrome the two main problems are:

1. *Tension in mooladhara chakra* related to deep unconscious fears such as fear of death, insecurity and losing possessions.
2. *Tension in manipura chakra*, which manifests as anxiety in people with irritable colon. This is one side of the coin which expresses itself either as anger and rage if directed outward, or as anxiety if directed inward. We can see this dual nature of the sympathetic nervous system's response to stress in the 'fight or flight' mechanism. When faced with stress we must choose to either stay and fight (rage) or fly (fear). People with irritable bowel syndrome are affected by the latter.

The sympathetic system of these people is very weak. It is usually taxed and strained by real and imaginary anxieties, fears, thoughts of past and future calamities, guilt, suppression, etc. so when the sufferer meets up with a truly stressful situation there is not enough strength and energy to cope. The sympathetic system fatigues quickly and stops working, resulting in overemphasis of the parasympathetic component and consequent speeding up of peristalsis and diarrhoea. If the sympathetic system regains strength, it suppresses motility and constipation sets in. So in the irritable bowel syndrome we see one or more of the following symptoms:

- Diarrhoea when the sympathetic system is fatigued and parasympathetic system is overactive.
- Constipation when the sympathetic system is dominating and the parasympathetic system is underactive.

- Alternating diarrhoea and constipation when the sympathetic system is not quite depleted of energy.

The essential starting point for the whole disease is dissipation of mind, body and energy. This lack of concentration and integrity allows the body mechanisms to fatigue and run without sufficient control. Thus the irritable bowel syndrome reflects our conscious or unconscious irritation with life as a whole and ourselves.

Overcoming the cause

The typical person with irritable bowels is a tense, conscientious individual who worries excessively about family or financial matters. These are basically good people who have taken on their own or other people's burdens with excessive seriousness and lack of insight. When they use meditation, karma yoga or other yogic techniques, they progress quite quickly by using the same mental attitude in a positive way. Tension is replaced by cheerfulness and the insight gained from yoga helps solve their problems.

The combination of medical science and yoga is a practical approach to this problem. Initially, a doctor can allay many fears, especially of cancer, by excluding the possibility of organic disease. For extreme tension in certain cases, tranquillizers may be used for a short time. However, in the majority of cases drugs have no comparison with yoga in terms of safety, efficacy and long term improvement.

Here are a few suggestions which will help you to understand and eliminate nervous diarrhoea:
- In most cases the diarrhoea is not severe and will not cause further disease in itself. It indicates that tensions within are being expelled and expressed via the physical medium. Though uncomfortable, it can be tolerated. If it becomes excessive and you feel a little dehydrated (dry tongue, decreased urine) drink extra water, fruit juice and other beverages.
- Diarrhoea is a high metabolic energy process in which there is a fast turnover of body cells, nutrition and so on.

129

The eliminative process is dominant over absorption and this tends to clean out impurities and toxins assimilated because of mental and physical tension and indiscretion etc. Some people say it is better than a fast.

- At the same time, diarrhoea is a gauge by which you can judge your physical condition. As your health improves, your stool will also become normal. Whenever you get an attack of nervous diarrhoea, watch the process in action and the thoughts that come to your mind. You can learn a lot about yourself in this way.
- Try to make a deep and sincere resolve to put all your effort into overcoming those things that cause you anxiety. In this way you gain a direction, a goal towards which you can aim your lifestyle and habits.
- Dietary measures often help, for example, increasing the roughage (fruits, raw vegetables, salad, bran, whole grains, etc.) for constipation, and decreasing it for diarrhoea.
- If the diarrhoea is excessive and causes you so much inconvenience that you cannot carry out your daily duties, then tincture of belladonna is suggested. This will remove pain and slow down the movement of the intestines. It is an old fashioned method but probably one of the best. Other remedies are kaolin, which is basically chalk, and atropine-based drugs such as Lomotil.
- Reassurance, knowledge of what the disease is all about, calming the emotions and the mind, and yogic sadhana are the best combination for treatment.

Nervous diarrhoea sadhana

This sadhana incorporates relaxation and practices designed to restabilize mooladhara and manipura chakras.

1. *Asana*: Pawanmuktasana parts 1 and 2, vajrasana (especially after meals, with breath awareness), shashank-asana, shavasana (with abdominal breath awareness).
2. *Pranayama*: Nadi shodhana (no retention), seetkari, bhramari.
3. *Meditation*: Yoga nidra, antar mouna, chidakasha dharana.

ACUTE DIARRHOEA

Acute diarrhoea is a medical problem, not a yogic one. However, it can be handled more effectively if yoga is used as an adjunct to medicine. Occasionally a yogi will find himself in a situation where he can use yoga to prevent a potentially serious case of diarrhoea from even starting. Acute diarrhoea can be due to any of the following:

- *Gastroenteritis,* inflammation of the whole digestive tract, in which diarrhoea usually occurs from one to 48 hours after the consumption of contaminated food or drink.
- *Specific infectious diseases* such as enteric fever, dysentery, or cholera which are spread by infected drinking water and food. They do not show up immediately after the consumption of food as their incubation period is longer than food poisoning.
- *Food allergy,* when the food ingested is wholesome, but the patient's reaction to it is abnormal. This is quite rare.
- *Digestive upsets* which result from eating food that is too rich, like fat, or irritating food such as unripe fruit.

Food poisoning

Gastroenteritis, the most common form of diarrhoea, can be caused by:

- *Poisonous foods* such as certain fungi and certain tropical fish.
- *Chemical poisoning,* for example, if a container has held poisons before food was placed in it, or if acid foods were kept in cheap enamel or zinc vessels liberating antimony or zinc. Other metals such as lead, mercury, arsenic and cadmium may also cause diarrhoea if ingested.
- *Bacterial poisoning,* which is divided into two main groups:
  i) The toxin type in which bacteria release toxins into the food. These bacteria usually come from an infected person handling the food. There is an infamous but rare form of this type of poisoning called *botulism,* which is very serious and usually fatal. It is caused by

131

certain bacteria in canned foods where there has been inefficient processing, and imperfectly preserved fish. The toxin produced is one of the most potent poisons known.

ii) The infectious type usually comes from the salmonella group, and less commonly from the paratyphoid and staphylococcal groups. Salmonella is usually transferred to food by an infected handler, flies, mice, excreta, etc. The types of food which are particularly likely to be infected are meat dishes, stews, gravies, soups, custards, milk, synthetic cream and tinned food. Outbreaks of food poisoning are especially likely to occur in hot weather when food is prepared for large numbers of people and the remaining food is saved for later without adequate storage facilities.

Note that food poisoning is usually found in more than one member of a family which helps to point out the cause of the infection.

The main symptoms of food poisoning are nausea, vomiting, diarrhoea and abdominal pain. If severe, the patient may collapse. Recovery usually takes place within 48 hours. The doctor must distinguish food poisoning from surgical conditions such as acute appendicitis, intestinal obstruction, intussuception and volvulus.

Treatment

Most cases of gastroenteritis are mild and can be treated at home with bed rest, warmth, care and love. Plenty of warm fluids such as fruit drinks and water with glucose should be taken to wash out poisons and prevent dehydration. No food should be taken until the condition improves and the appetite returns. At this stage give a semi-fluid, low roughage diet, including barley water with a little sugar or salt, white bread or toast, white rice, fruit juice, boiled green banana and rice, or plain curd (yoghurt) and rice. Heat applied to the abdomen is also helpful.

Vomiting may be stopped by anti-vomiting drugs such as Stemetil; if it continues unabated, it becomes dry retching and constitutes a threat to the organism. As a rule vomiting and diarrhoea are left to continue their natural course as they are the body's way of removing the poisons in the shortest possible time.

Antibiotics are not recommended for the typical case of food poisoning as they tend to prolong the disorder rather than cure it. The milder conditions are self-limiting, that is, they cure themselves. Typhoid, cholera, and the more severe forms are treated with antibiotics of the doctor's choice. A competent doctor is required to differentiate mild poisoning from severe, and to distinguish food poisoning from digestive upsets caused by excess sweets, fats, etc.

Yogic prevention and therapy

By eliminating excessive or upsetting foods, or those containing poisonous or infectious bacteria from the stomach before they can act on the body, we can effectively stop acute diarrhoea in its tracks. The yogic technique vyaghra kriya accomplishes this. Using warm salty water, vomiting is induced as many times as is required to completely clean the stomach. In this way poisons do not travel to the intestines for absorption into the bloodstream. At the same time prana is generated in the manipura chakra area, increasing strength and vitality.

During the illness, shavasana with abdominal breath awareness, yoga nidra and antar mouna can be used to allow the natural cleansing and defensive processes to go on unimpeded. If there is no fever, kunjal kriya can be performed to reduce nausea. As there is a chance that this may induce a mild rise in body temperature because of its action on manipura chakra (the solar plexus), a bath should not be taken until three hours after performing kunjal. Immediately after kunjal is finished, rest for 20 minutes then drink some warm liquids to replace fluid loss. After this try to sleep as much as possible. Usually, though, once the acute illness has set in, yoga is out.

133

CHRONIC DIARRHOEA

This is not a disease in itself but a symptom of many diseases and disorders. Chronic diarrhoea in western countries is usually due to nervous diarrhoea, cancer of the colon, diverticulitis, ulcerative colitis, and other post-operative effects. Other factors must also be considered: bacteria, worms, protozoa, etc. If there is an infection and/or ulceration, there is usually pain. Cancer of the colon is usually painless unless it obstructs the flow of faeces. It often occurs in the elderly, so people in this age group are advised to have a regular medical check-up. Blood and mucus in the stool is usually a sign of dysentery, not diarrhoea, but they can also be found in the stools of those who have cancer.

Anyone with chronic diarrhoea or dysentery should contact a doctor and have a thorough check-up. The exact cause of the illness must be discovered and only if medical advice is completely unobtainable should self-medication be undertaken.

Dysentery

This is inflammation of the colon and rectum which is characterized by abdominal pain and the passage of frequent stools containing blood and mucus. It is caused by bacteria and protozoa such as amoeba. There are two kinds of dysentery:

1. *Bacilliary dysentery* is caused by the genus shigella. They are found all over the world, and are seen in epidemics wherever there is a large population with poor sanitation. In the tropics it is spread by flies and also from person to person because of hands being inadequately washed. Outbreaks are common in institutions. Sometimes bacilliary dysentery is so mild that it is hardly noticeable as it only consists of a few loose stools and a little pain. Other times it is so severe that death can occur within 48 hours, although this is rare.

2. *Amoebic dysentery* is usually a disease with little or no fever, and in this way differs from bacilliary dysentery which is an acute disease associated with fever. It causes ulceration of the wall of the colon and can spread to the liver where it will cause an abscess. The symptoms of this disease are usually grumbling stomach and pains in the abdomen. There are usually two or more loose stools per day, and periods of diarrhoea alternating with constipation occur. Mucus is often passed and the stools have a most offensive odour. The abdomen is usually tender, especially over the line of the colon.

Treatment

Dysentery is generally treated with bed rest (which also prevents this disease from spreading), plenty of fluids, a semi-fluid and low roughage diet, and drugs. The following suggestions are also helpful:

- Fast for one day, drinking only water with glucose or fresh citrus fruit juices as you feel the need.
- For one week take psyllium husks (Isabgol) and curd mixed with water three or four times throughout the day. The curd replaces harmful bacteria with beneficial bacteria that reline the intestinal wall and help to cut down the infection. Because they are not digested, the psyllium husks move through the system like a vacuum cleaner.
- After a week, return to a light diet, mainly consisting of boiled green bananas, boiled rice and curd (yoghurt). Continue this for a few days and gradually bring yourself back to a normal diet, with the emphasis on individual needs.

If you wish to attempt the removal of chronic dysentery using yogic techniques you should contact a skilled yoga therapist. In chronic amoebic dysentery, shankhaprakshalana can be used, but only with great care. It may be combined with fasting, kunjal and neti, asanas and pranayama selected for each individual case, yoga nidra and prana vidya. A skilled yoga teacher or therapist can bring the body back to sound health, especially when working in conjunction with a sympathetic physician.

Colitis

Other common causes of chronic diarrhoea, especially in the west, are ulcerative colitis and Crohn's disease. These conditions occur most commonly in those between the ages of 20 to 40 years and the main symptoms are loose bloody stool with mucus, pain and tenderness in the abdomen, fever, tachycardia and exhaustion.

Medically speaking the organic cause is unknown, though certain theories are given:
- An auto-immune process is at work in which the body becomes allergic to its own tissues and in this case the colon becomes involved.
- Hypersensitivity to certain foods exists. This, however, is not really an accepted theory.
- It is psychological in origin, as seen in people who tend to have undue dependence on others, extreme sensitivity to personal slights and obsessive tendencies. Though this theory is widely accepted, medical science is not certain whether it is causative or an effect of the disease.

From the yogic point of view, colitis has deep mental roots. People with colitis usually have an indefinite aim in life and are prone to frequent feelings of hopelessness and of helplessness. This is basically due to imbalance in the mooladhara chakra, a disturbance in the self-preservation instinct. Yoga has the means to approach the root of this problem and to eradicate it.

Medical therapy consists of such measures as hospital admission in severe cases and drug therapy. Tranquillizers may also be used for anxiety and agitation, which are both causative and aggravating factors. The course of the illness is one of exacerbation and remission, becoming particularly bad when the unconscious material from mooladhara chakra is surfacing most actively and disappearing when the mind has become content, happy and peaceful.

136

It is with this in mind that yoga deals with the problems of colitis. Meditation techniques are particularly useful in helping to handle the surfacing material. They also offer more insight into life and thus help us to choose a suitable purpose and direction by overcoming the helpless, hopeless factor.

Colitis sadhana

The following practices, when learned under expert guidance, are useful in relieving the distressing symptoms, eventually bringing about cure and, if practised regularly, they help to prevent relapse.

1. *Hatha yoga shatkriya*: Laghoo shankhaprakshalana, moola shodhana, basti.
2. *Asana*: Pawanmuktasana (part 1 for severe cases and part 2 for mild cases), vajrasana (after meals with breath awareness), shavasana (with awareness of abdominal breath).
3. *Pranayama*: Nadi shodhana, bhramari, ujjayi.
4. *Meditation*: Yoga nidra, antar mouna, chidakasha dharana, ajapa japa.

Yogic adjuncts

During a bout of chronic diarrhoea or dysentery, certain techniques can be used to relax the source of tension and relieve pain. Remembrance of God, guru or mantra is very powerful. It can also take the form of visualization, perhaps a special symbol, a peaceful scene, a healing colour. The practice of pure awareness, watching the body, breath and mind, and the various responses to the illness are also recommended. Antar mouna allows the thoughts, visions and feelings of the subconscious, many of which cause inner tension, weakening the body and mind, to surface and be eliminated. Yoga nidra completely relaxes the body-mind, relieves pain and conserves energy.

During the period of convalescence, pawanmuktasana and mild nadi shodhana help to rebalance the energies of the body. Meditation practices such as yoga nidra, antar mouna, chidakasha dharana and japa relax the mind and quell any turbulence in the body. Later, as convalescence progresses, hatha yoga shatkarmas act directly on the digestive system purifying and strengthening it.

PREVENTION

General preventive measures

In terms of diarrhoea and dysentery, the following measures will help to maintain good health wherever sanitation and hygiene are a problem.

- All drinking water should be boiled and then kept in a previously boiled bottle.
- All milk should be boiled.
- All food should be well cooked, recently cooked and cooked only once.
- All fruit which is not cooked should be peeled or washed in a little clean water.
- Do not eat food which has been cooked previously and left out uncovered.
- Avoid fly infested restaurants. If the dining room has flies, the kitchen will have more. If the restaurant toilet is dirty, the kitchen will also be dirty.
- To prevent poisoning, great care should be taken with the preparation of food so that it is free of contaminated contents. Food that is left over for future use should always be covered and kept in a cool place. This will keep away flies and prevent bacteria from multiplying.
- In hot climates and during summer, more care should be taken. People with cuts or sores on their hands should not touch food that is to be eaten.
- Yogic cleansing techniques help to eliminate harmful bacteria from the digestive tract.
- Yogic practices in general will increase the body's resistance, thereby reducing the tendency for bacterial diseases such as dysentery to occur.

Yogic prevention

A dichotomy in terms of world health has arisen. Western countries emphasize outer cleanliness and prevention of bacterial spread, but they have not yet stressed the importance of the mind in preventing disease – the 'constitution factor'. In the East the opposite situation exists – the mind is given first priority, ignoring the infectious agent. As a result, infectious diseases are rampant in the East, while psychosomatic diseases are rampant in the West. Obviously some meeting point must be reached. People in the West need to improve their constitutional and mental health as much as people in the East need to improve sanitation and hygiene. In this way, diseases such as peptic ulcer, on the one hand, and amoebic dysentery, on the other, will cease to pose such a threat.

Yoga is the obvious solution to both these problems. It makes us more aware and sensitive to our inner needs and the needs of our environment, which are ultimately one and the same. Regular practice is the means to improve our physical, emotional and mental health. Yoga channels our energies, making them useful, creative, purposeful and practical rather than disease-producing and destructive. Our energies can be channelled both internally and externally. Along with daily practices, karma yoga, bhakti yoga and jnana yoga help us to improve ourselves and the world around us.

Our state of being has a powerful effect on the environment. As our own lifestyle becomes more simple, clean and ordered, we tend to make our immediate surroundings the same also. Family and friends are quick to notice the positive change and may also be inspired to improve themselves. The yogic process of increasing health and mental peace is infectious and leads to prevention of disease on a long term and world-wide basis.

18

Obesity

Obesity is undoubtedly the most common medical problem in many countries. It is important to reduce obesity as it shortens the lifespan, lowers the efficiency of all the bodily organs and detracts from the ability to participate in normal activities. Moreover, many diseases are associated with obesity: diabetes, osteoarthritis, gout, hernia, varicose veins, bronchitis, skin infections, gall stones, arteriosclerosis, hypertension, angina pectoris and cardiac failure.

Most people consider the typical obese person to be a big, round, jolly fellow continually pushing food down a throat covered with three or four double chins. This picture, however, is far from the truth. Most obese people are not at all jolly and the majority do not even consider themselves to be obese. Due to social pressures they often feel inferior and isolated because of society's ideal image of a trim athletic body.

Medically speaking, obesity is the presence of surplus body fat and it is defined as weight greater than 20 pounds over the average for height and age. Obesity only applies to fat and not to muscle and bone. For example, the extra weight an athlete puts on is not obesity but is due to extra muscle bulk, called muscular hypertrophy.

Beneath the surface

Obesity is caused mainly through overeating and lack of exercise but these have as their basis many cultural, social and psychological factors. The tendency towards obesity depends to a degree on genetic and racial predisposition. Geographical, climatic, occupational and the rural or urban nature of the environment determine the severity and prevalence. Traditions, habits, and access to servants or modern conveniences which eliminate the need for physical work are all contributing factors. Physiological causes such as damage to the brain centres controlling hunger and glandular imbalance are rare and considered less important on average.

Perhaps the basic psychological component is a low sense of self-esteem coupled with an unconscious problem of personal identity. These lead to feelings of emptiness and insecurity and the need to stuff the body with food in the hope of making it more solid, real and secure. The longing that results from frustration of pleasure, power, or affection leads people to fill up on food in order to feel more complete. Some people eat because of 'mouth hunger'. Though they have no desire to put anything in their stomachs, they require something in their mouth. For others, food becomes a narcotic, a means to escape the boredom and tension of life. Many use food to stop the gnawing pain of anxiety, mistakenly identified as hunger.

The mental tensions that cause obesity have many different origins in the unconscious mind. Try to see what mechanisms cause you and others around you to overeat and get fat. Yoga techniques will help you to explore your inner nature and discover them.

Fat research

It is thought by some that fatness depends on the number of fat cells in the body. These cells are like bags which store fat. They increase in number only during childhood and adolescence, but not in adulthood. Rats which were overfed during early growth were compared with underfed rats. When both groups were placed on a normal diet, the overfed continued to stay obese.[1] This implies that obese children

141

have less chance of losing excess fat than those people who become obese later in life. It is postulated that this is because, when the fat cells deflate they trigger the hunger centres in the hypothalamus, imitating chronic hunger, and therefore we gain weight again. If this theory proves to be true, it should be remembered that yoga offers the means to effectively remedy this cellular imbalance at both the structural and functional levels. To prevent chronic obesity parents should be careful not to overfeed their children lest they suffer the consequences.

Other studies show that obese people have a characteristic behaviour that differs from normal.[2] Obese people are thought to be unable to differentiate internal cues commonly thought to regulate appetite. For example, fear suppresses appetite in normal people but enhances it in the obese. Environmental cues such as smell, sight or taste of food, the sight of other people eating and the time of day affect the behaviour of obese people more.

Metabolism

Why is it that some people feel more hungry than others? Why is it that some people can eat and eat without getting fat even though they are relatively inactive, while others who are a little more active can put on weight with just a morsel of food? The answer lies between the body and mind in the flow of energies.

The body functions on the dual basis of input and output. This is metabolism, "the sum of all the physical and chemical processes by which living, organized substance is produced and maintained (anabolism) and also the transformation by which energy is made available for the uses of the organism (catabolism)."[3] In normal people, energies 'in' balance those 'out' so that stable, healthy weight is maintained. However, obese individuals take in more than they put out.

Because of mental tensions that cause craving and addiction to food, our neuroendocrine systems become unbalanced and the metabolism is thrown into disequilibrium. This may result in a greater build-up than breakdown of fat. The tendency to overeat may occur in either of two states:

1. A high energy state in which energy utilization is the same as or a little more than calorie intake.
2. A low energy state in which calorie intake is greater than energy utilization.

In yoga we say that people in a high energy state are rajasic while those in a low energy state are tamasic. The balanced, healthy state is sattwic. Both tamasic and rajasic people like to eat, and usually in large quantities. Rajasic people who are active and dynamic, and whose desire is channelled into activity through ambition, need to eat a lot and to eat the things they like. They do not usually become obese, however, because they burn up the energy in work and activity. Tamasic people, on the other hand, often eat out of boredom or to forget themselves and the world around them. These people like leisure, pleasure and just lying around. For them eating is a better pastime than working, but because they are not active they do not burn up the fuel. They like to do little more than just eating and sleeping.

Sattwic people derive most of their energy from a higher source and see food in its correct perspective, as a means to provide fuel and building blocks for the body. Thus they may eat much or little, depending on what the body needs. They know how to work hard with full concentration and how to relax with full awareness. They work with an attitude of karma yoga (selfless service); their hearts are full of bhakti (devotion to the higher forces and humanity), and their minds are immersed in jnana (knowledge of the fundamentals of life and existence). Sattwic individuals are aware, free and open to all aspects of life. They can eat what they like because with awareness they appreciate things that are wholesome and good for them. This is the outcome of the yogic balancing and reintegrating process.

143

Yogic approach to reducing

Yoga tackles obesity from two main directions. The first approach is to rebalance the metabolic process. The second is to release unconscious personality blocks and complexes, for example, to show people that they are not as bad as they think themselves to be.

It is possible through yoga to completely restructure the subtle pranic body to affect the metabolic turnover of energy. While doing this, efforts are also made to directly alter the reactivity of the hunger and satiety centres in the hypothalamus. Overexcitement of the hunger centre and insensitivity of the satiety centre must be rebalanced and pulled in opposite directions. This tightening has an effect on the whole body, making it more compact and slim. Thus, even though we may have more fat cells than normal, by attacking the problem centrally in the brain rather than peripherally in the fat cells, we can readjust the body's tone and effectively reduce the pull of fat cells on the brain to feed them.

Internal sensitivity results from refining the nervous system and the pranic components of the body. By relaxing the mind, we calm the nerves and make them both less reactive to outside stimuli and more reactive to inner cues. We must be careful when we attempt such a reintegrative process because it is necessary to know which way to turn the control, whether up or down. For example, the practice of bhastrika pranayama increases our appetite and burns up food through the increased fire of metabolism, while meditation decreases appetite and craving and also lowers the metabolic rate. A balanced approach is required so that the metabolic fire in the obese person is enhanced but the emotional tension is not increased. Only an experienced guide can help you with this.

Note that many people with a sluggish metabolism may appear to be a little overweight without necessarily suffering from obesity. Often people think they are too fat, when they really are not. Therefore, before you start to treat yourself for a weight problem, be sure that it really exists.

Helpful hints

When trying to reduce excess fat, it is important not to attempt too much or to expect results too quickly. It takes time to put on weight and so it also takes time to take it off, especially if we wish to keep it off. Sometimes weight loss is rapid in the first few weeks as water is being eliminated. Then the initial progress slows and excitement gives way to impatience, disappointment and discouragement. Severe depression may set in if the person is not adequately informed about these facts. A steady weight loss of one to two pounds (½–1 kilogram) per week should be attempted.

Drugs and fad diets are not useful in the long term. Fad diets may quickly reduce the weight, but because the body and brain do not have time to adjust, chronic hunger results and weight quickly comes back. Also they do not resolve the emotional factor and they may be nutritionally deficient.

It is far better to eat two or three meals per day of regular amounts and at regular times so as to break external cues. At the same time eliminate all snack and processed foods which increase calories and decrease vitality. As a rule, food should not be taken while watching television, reading or talking, as these activities deprive you of the full satisfaction of eating and thus tend to induce continued eating.

Total abstinence, the classical treatment for some addictions, is not feasible in the case of food. Also, do not feel guilty about occasional overindulgences. These do not hurt us really, but the guilt can lead to a period of fasting, followed up with increased hunger, craving and then more overindulgence. The constant seesaw of body weight, due to alternate dieting and indulgence, disturbs the body's metabolism and the neuro-endocrine balance.

Until your body and mind have adjusted to new dietary habits, it is best to eat what you like, even 'forbidden' foods such as chocolate, pastries, chips, etc. but only eat a little. At the same time, make a diet of whole foods for yourself that you can live with for your daily life, and have this as the basis for all food intake.

Be sure to get plenty of physical exercise. Give more time to housework, gardening, sports and yoga. A 30 minute walk each day will also help, especially after meals. The more active you are the less time you will have to think about food.

Forget food and live life

The simplest and also the best cure for obesity is to experience the joy of living. Many people live life from an armchair; they prefer to watch and observe rather than participate actively. They fill themselves with all the nutrients necessary for active healthy living, but they never burn them up. Thus the mind and body become clogged and constipated, the metabolism sluggish, and fat deposits itself. When people become fat, they naturally feel self-conscious and project their complex onto their favourite subject, food. As a result, even though they want to lose weight, their thoughts are always with food. Constantly thinking about eating or not eating is called a food neurosis. While food is so much a part of one's mind and life it is not possible to lose weight. The only way is to busy the mind in other pursuits.

You can redirect your thoughts by making a sankalpa or resolve such as "I will become slim and active". See yourself each morning as you wake up, happy, alert and thin. Move into each day with a positive and dynamic attitude. Immerse yourself in karma yoga, and work with a relaxed and free mind. Become busy with life, participate, engage yourself, do not be afraid to utilize your resources. Be creative, everyone has inherent talents and abilities, although they may need to be brought out and developed. Live life to the fullest and the satisfaction you will gain will more than satisfy your hunger. Your need for excess food will spontaneously diminish as your other needs are met.

Obesity sadhana

The following program helps to reduce obesity by stabilizing the metabolism and removing the underlying emotional

146

problems. It should ideally follow a full course of shankha-prakshalana, which helps the process by eliminating toxins and speeding up a sluggish metabolism.

1. *Hatha yoga shatkriya*: Laghoo shankhaprakshalana, kunjal and neti, agnisar and nauli.
2. *Asana*: Surya namaskara (up to a maximum of 108 rounds, building up gradually over a period of months), pawan-muktasana part 2.
3. *Pranayama*: Bhastrika.
4. *Meditation*: Any technique.

Yoga improves concentration, willpower and helps us to realize our potential. Through meditation we reduce our craving for any outside means of satisfying our inner insecurity, and we begin to free ourselves from their grasp on us. At the same time we begin to see and hear inside and therefore can discriminate where our hunger is coming from, whether from the mind, the stomach, the tongue or the genitals. Then we can eat what we need and when we need it, while satisfying our other urges appropriately.

19

Poor Nutrition

Have you ever gone hungry? Real hunger to the point of starvation is fortunately a rare experience for most of us. However, statistics show that at least 300 million children in the world experience malnutrition and even starvation every day and perhaps very rarely satisfy it. In fact, half the people in the world today are protein deficient. The dichotomy between 'East' and 'West' becomes obvious when we realize just how unevenly distributed the world's food resources are. This imbalance is reflected in the diseases of excess so prevalent in the West, and of poor nutrition so common in the East.

Poor nutrition is basically of two types:
1. *Undernutrition* – not enough food, and
2. *Malnutrition* – the wrong sort of food

Poor nutrition can be due to physical or mental factors. In the East it is mainly caused by food shortage and the high price of foodstuffs in proportion to the average daily wage. Another cause of poor nutrition is chronic amoebic dysentery, worms and other intestinal parasites. In the West it occurs because of an unbalanced diet containing too many highly processed foods, or psychological factors. Other causes to be decided by a doctor are cancer of the stomach, persistent vomiting and alcohol (which adds calories but leads to malnutrition).

Undernutrition

Severe malnutrition in countries sapped by chronic food shortages due to war, flood and famine is a well-known picture to most people. Malnutrition, however, has further implications in long term undernutrition, affecting millions of children for the rest of their lives.

The brain requires a steady and adequate supply of nutrients, not only for maintenance but to ensure correct functioning. Food provides the building blocks without which the brain cannot build its complex interconnected neuronal circuits and switches. According to J. Dobbing and J. Sands of the University of Manchester, England, brain growth has two phases: the first prenatal phase is the stage of initial growth and formation of cells for which nutrition comes from the mother constantly. The second is postnatal and is called the 'brain growth spurt'. This is the most vulnerable period in development during which inadequate nutrition and lack of nutrition inflict lasting damage.[1] Their research shows that more than 80% of the growth spurt occurs after birth.

It is not the number of cells which are affected by nutrition but their organization. Particularly vulnerable to poor nutrition is the cerebellum which appears to actually weigh less in undernourished rats as compared to normally fed ones. This may explain the poor coordination, clumsiness and reduced manual skills in malnourished children. B.G. Cragg from Monash University, Australia, found that rats malnourished early in life have up to 40% reduction in the number of minute nerve endings in the brain's cortex.[2] He also found molecular breaks in some nerve endings and postulated that they, therefore, would not function.

Roger Lewin points out that: "If the undernourished cerebral cortex really lacks almost half of its interconnections (or even one tenth), the consequences for brain function are frightening. The planet may be raising a generation of clumsy, feeble-minded millions."[3] He goes on to state that moderate degrees of malnutrition, which 300 million children

149

experience daily, can produce these effects. Normal feeding does not completely remedy the damage, though it improves the grosser aspects of development; language development and verbal concept formation suffer, for example. Physically, smaller stature, lighter weight and smaller heads than normal may develop in the malnourished. Behaviourally, these children do not do as well at school and are generally somewhat disadvantaged.

Nutritional inadequacy must be kept in perspective with the lack of environmental stimulation that most of these malnourished children suffer. It is a well known fact that poor stimulation leads to mental starvation. Stephen Richardson and his colleagues showed that a nutritious diet plus mental stimulation are both necessary for intelligence.[4] Among well nourished, healthy children, those from a stimulating environment did better than those from a poor environment. These in turn did better then malnourished children. Of malnourished children, those in stimulating environments did better in intelligence tests than those from a poor environment.

To overcome the problem of poor nutrition the first priority must go to food, then yoga can be used to enhance brain development and potential. Prevention, of course, is always best, especially with children. Adolfo Chavez from Mexico found that when children are well nourished before and after birth, they are healthier physically, have superior language development, are more active and vigorous in play, more independent and exploratory.[5] Therefore, their parents and siblings take more interest in them and provide more stimulus.

When the damage has been done, much can still be remedied in terms of compensating for the basic deficit, as shown by Leonardo Sinisterra in Cali, Colombia.[6] Giving "massive doses of good diet, fun and games, teaching and stimulation can help to overcome the intelligence gap that malnutrition leaves in its wake"[7] We have also found that children placed in the ashram environment thrive on the yogic diet and the high level of stimulation and creativity. Within a few months they become markedly brighter, sharper and quicker than other children of the same age group.

By now, some of you may be wondering whether you would have been more intelligent if your parents had known about these things. If this question should arise, it is good to remember that yoga has the answer. Science is now proving that yoga can support the restructure of the cortex of the brain. The effects of early deprivation do not have to be permanent, even at a late stage in life if you have the determination to increase your awareness and brain capacity through yogic techniques. Food is important, but a scientific method such as yoga, which stimulates and activates both brain and body, may be a boon for all those who have suffered from the double insult of poverty – a dearth of food and unstimulating environmental conditions.

Malnutrition

Any diet deficient in the correct balance of proteins, vitamins, minerals, etc. leads to malnutrition. Examples of malnutrition are kwashiorkor (protein deficiency caused by displacing the child from the breast when the next child is born), marasamus (protein plus calorie deficiency), night blindness (vitamin A deficiency), rickets (vitamin D deficiency), blood clotting disorders (vitamin K deficiency), scurvy (vitamin C deficiency), beri beri (vitamin B_1 deficiency) and pellagra (niacin deficency).

The obvious cure for these conditions is to replace the deficiency. However, it is only in the last 50 years that doctors have realized that diseases might be due to lack of some essential factor. When this concept was recognized, a revolution took place in medical thought. The nutritional diseases which were rampant within the lifetime of some doctors still practising have now vanished under the affluence of technology. For example, in the United Kingdom, florid rickets is a clinical curiosity though many carry the scars of

151

it. In southern USA pellagra affected tens of thousands of people before 1940 and is now scarcely heard of.

By supplying the correct amount of calories and nutrients these nutritional diseases are eradicated. The minimum calorie intake required by the UK Department of Health and Social Security is 3000 per day for a man and 2200 for a woman.

Malnutrition and weight loss are also common in gastrointestinal disease. This is generally due to a reduced food intake because of anorexia (loss of appetite), nausea or vomiting, but it can also be caused by poor absorption of nutrients or loss of protein from a diseased bowel as in dysentery or ulcerative colitis. Amoebic dysentery is a huge problem in may parts of the world, leading to chronic disability. Even after successful drug therapy, reinfection is common. Therapy for these conditions must include drugs, education in food preparation, hygiene, sanitation and methods of increasing constitutional strength through yogic practices.

Psychological problems

Fear, worry and other chronic tensions may manifest as loss of appetite and therefore underweight. When our mind is full of conflict, food does not taste good. Psychological tension and anxiety may also manifest as worry about being too thin. This worry itself often causes further tension, loss of appetite, decreased food intake, making one even thinner. Worry about being too fat, on the other hand, may lead to anorexia nervosa, an extreme condition in which fasting is carried to the point of starvation, yet the deluded individual still fears that he or she is too fat.

Constitutional factor

Some people are not constitutionally meant to be large muscled or fat. People who are thin by nature are called ectomorphs; they are genetically programmed to have small bones and a slight build. They differ from the muscle bound mesomorph and the fat endomorph in that they do not put on weight easily. Being prone to excessive thinking and brooding, ectomorphs have a highly developed nervous system built for mental work, but a less developed muscular and digestive system. Any imbalance makes them thinner and physically debilitated so that they tend to look weaker than they really are.

For those who are constitutionally ectomorphic or who are suffering from psychological problems which keep them thin, a yogic sadhana can be devised which will have far more long-term benefits than traditional body building exercises. The true ectomorph who seeks increased body size through various muscle building techniques may even sacrifice mental strength for the extra muscle bulk gained in this way. Real strength lies in coordinating body and mind, in willpower and awareness, not just in large muscles which are associated with hard physical labour. Through yoga we learn to focus our energies and find that we are more than just our physical body.

Underweight sadhana

Yogasanas are an excellent way to increase body strength and agility, for they tone muscles and teach coordination. Pranayama awakens the energy and helps to fan the gastric fire at manipura chakra. Meditation increases mental strength through relaxation and concentration, thereby revealing the all-powerful light of the spirit.

Here are some specific techniques which the underweight person may find very useful.
1. *Hatha yoga shatkriya*: Shankhaprakshalana and laghoo shankhaprakshalana, kunjal and neti.
2. *Asana*: Surya namaskara, pawanmuktasana, paschimottanasana, dhanurasana, sarvangasana, ardha matsyendrasana.
3. *Pranayama*: Bhastrika, nadi shodhana, ujjayi.
4. *Meditation*: Ajapa japa, kriya yoga.

20

Diet and Disease

Cancer, arthritis, asthma, heart disease and many more other degenerative conditions are now being related to dietary intake. Not only this, but the various relatively simple digestive upsets are seen by many experts to be just the first step in the long degenerative descent.

In 1977 the USA Senate Select Committee on Nutrition and Human Needs released an 85-page report in which they stated that: "During this century, the composition of the average diet has changed radically. Complex carbohydrates, fruits, vegetables, and grain products which were the mainstay of the diet, now play a minority role. At the same time, fat and sugar consumption have risen to the point where these dietary elements alone now comprise at least 60% of the total caloric intake, an increase of 20% since the early 1900s... These and other changes in the diet... may be as profoundly damaging to the nation's health as the widespread contagious diseases of the early part of the century."[1] This report links diet to six of the ten leading causes of death, including cancer.

Cancer

In the light of recent scientific discoveries, the link between diet and cancer has been recognized and widely accepted. Many experts are even stating that nutrition is one of the major factors in the cause, prevention and permanent cure of cancer. Dr G.B. Gori, Deputy of the National Cancer Institute Division of Cancer Cause and Prevention (USA), has stated: "Epidemiologic (environmental) and laboratory data suggests that diet is an important factor in the causation of various forms of cancer... improper diet is related to 60% of all cancers in men and 41% in women."[2]

Some authorities state that it is the cancer-causing substances contained in food which are responsible, while others state that the actual proportions of food intake, the quality and way it is eaten are more important. Probably both are concomitant in their effects. For example, meat is said to contain many hormones, dyes and other chemicals with the potential to cause cancer. Dr B.K. Armstrong of the University of Western Australia has found that women on a vegetarian diet have a 30% lower mortality rate from breast cancer and 40% less uterine cancer than women who eat meat. Regarding the importance of the correct quantity of food, Dr Gori has stated that "of all dietary modifications, caloric restriction... with a few exceptions, generally inhibits tumour formation."[3] That is, if we eat less than the excessive amounts we have come to consider 'normal', then we have less likelihood of contracting cancer.

The link between diet and cancer is further illustrated by the experience of former movie star, Gloria Swanson. In the 1940s she was diagnosed as having uterine cancer and doctors recommended immediate surgery to remove her womb. Reluctant to take such measures, Miss Swanson consulted a nutritionist and on his advice adopted a wholefood diet consisting of grains, vegetables, a little fruit, and no animal protein. She also ate less, and 2 ½ years later tests showed her tumour had completely disappeared.

At this ashram we have seen many people who have used yoga, diet and willpower to overcome cancer. One 64-year-old woman who stayed with us was diagnosed as having cancer of the right kidney and was given less than one year to live. She changed her diet to vegetables, fruit and whole wheat bread only, and this, combined with a yogic lifestyle, gave her the good health and enthusiasm to travel around the world without difficulty.

The consumption of 'empty calories' in the form of processed, artificially flavoured and coloured foods made with white sugar and white flour also contributes to degenerative diseases. By eating meals based on these synthetic foods, people fail to eat adequate amounts of wholegrains and vegetables. Thus we find that people in affluent countries are eating too much but are actually suffering from just another form of malnutrition. Despite their prosperity, these people are literally starving themselves of good nourishing food. They may also be laying themselves open to cancer for natural foods are necessary for the maintenance of the body's systems, including the immunological mechanism that kills cancer cells before they can multiply and spread.

Heart disease

It has long been a controversial topic as to whether cholesterol is responsible for arteriosclerosis or hardening of the arteries. Cholesterol is a fatty substance manufactured in the body and taken in through the food we eat. When there is excessive absorption and internal production of cholesterol, this fat accumulates in the body and in the process of circulation it sticks to the blood vessels. This causes them to constrict and prevents the blood from reaching its destination. To compensate the heart must work harder, under greater pressure to pump the blood, and this leads to heart attack, hypertension and other vascular diseases.

Meat is the main source of cholesterol in the diet, followed by dairy products. Animal fats are called 'saturated' and have a high affinity for storage in the human body. Saturated fats are visible in meat and dairy products and invisible in cakes, pastries, thick soups and most cheeses. Eggs, butter and hard margarines are also full of saturated fats. It stands to reason that anyone with a heart problem should avoid saturated fats by reducing their intake of these foods. Dietary

156

restrictions combined with a less competitive and stressful lifestyle, and regular practice of yogic techniques, is an effective means of combating heart disease.

Arthritis

Perhaps the most interesting work on arthritis and diet was done by Eugene Dong, an American born Chinese doctor. After finishing his medical training he was almost crippled by arthritis. When every rheumatologist failed to remedy his condition he started to examine the question of diet. Inspired by the old Chinese adage: "All illnesses enter through the mouth", he changed his adopted American diet of hamburgers, orange juice, ice cream, etc. to rice, vegetables, seafood and a few other basic components of the traditional Chinese diet. He describes his cure as taking only a few short weeks.

From this experience, Dr Dong developed a theory in which he says that each body develops mechanisms to deal with its environment. For example, if you are of Western European or Scandinavian descent, it will be from 92 to 98% certain that you will be able to digest milk reasonably well. However, Greek, Cypriot, Jewish or Negroid blood will make the chances as high as 60 to 80% that you will not be able to digest milk or milk products satisfactorily. The plentiful supply of oranges in Mediterranean countries makes them perfect food for these peoples, while these same would be a form of poison to their Northern Scandinavian brothers. Apples, on the other hand, which grow in Scandinavia, would be the best fruit for these cold country dwellers. According to the experience of Dr Dong, red meat, sugar, milk and fruit (especially citrus) should be eliminated from the diet.

Dr Dong's work can be used to develop a base line for the appropriate diet for each environment and to best suit individual needs. In this way, we may avoid poisoning our systems with foods which we are not designed to handle, thus preventing such diseases as arthritis, cancer and heart disease. The whole question of the body's 'allergy' to certain foods, its inability to process some and its ability to process others is yet to be fully determined. However, this may prove to be one of the most challenging questions facing dietetics today.

Role of diet

Wrong diet is only one factor in the process of degeneration and disease. Tensions at all levels must be taken into account and eliminated to reverse the disease process. When we recognize the role of diet and mental tension, it will be possible to shortcircuit the downward process and actually prevent serious chronic conditions from occurring. When digestive disorders such as dyspepsia, diarrhoea, wind or constipation actually arise we can find through yoga, combined with other healing methods, a way to prevent their snowballing from relatively simple and easily treatable conditions into long-term disease beyond our reclamation.

It is the hope of yogis and healers that the role of diet in disease will be resolved or some practical directions given by science and the medical world, then the need for dietary restrictions would be more acceptable. Yoga has recognized this need and has combined dietary measures with its other techniques in an effort to reduce and eliminate the disease process. Through yoga we can examine our old food values and eating habits so as to better understand why we are eating certain foods and their effects on us. This understanding, which stems from increasing awareness, is the best way to solve the problem of diet related diseases and to see how diet can be used to increase health and general wellbeing.

21

Commentary on Diet

Discussion with Dr Swami Vivekananda
& Dr Swami Shankardevananda

Dr Swami Vivekananda: In the West you get a mixed audience of people, some who are into beverages, cups of coffee, plenty of meat and the whole typically western diet, while others are into very fine vegetarian diets. So, you have to take everyone from where they stand.

I was asked to do a whole day seminar on diet and declined because people get too involved in diet and it takes their attention away from the other possibilities of yoga. However, I do give a lecture in which I highlight various aspects of diet and give general guidelines as to how we should approach diet and what our attitude should be. The following chart is the basis of this lecture.

The horizontal axis shows the degree of cooking and processing, while the vertical axis represents the various types of foodstuff in descending, progressively heavier order, fruits being the lightest food and meat the heaviest food to digest. Junk food is really a non-food in that it has no intrinsic food value but is put on the list because so many people are eating these kinds of foods nowadays.

Most people in the West today are eating foods which fall into the synthetic junk food category (see lower and right side of chart), that is, mainly meat and processed and preserved food. Yogis, however, eat light food (see upper left corner of the chart). The ashram diet, for example, is mainly lightly cooked grains, legumes and vegetables and very occasionally fruit. Some yogis, of course eat only fruit and milk, which puts them up in the extreme left hand corner of this chart. However, this does not seem desirable for most people.

On a fruitarian diet you become so sensitive that you cannot really live a normal life. A disciple of Swami Satyananda's who used to live in San Francisco was taking this fruitarian diet and he had to leave San Francisco because he couldn't handle the noise of cars and so on. He went to live in a little town on the border of Oregon. Eventually, he felt this was too much for him, so now he lives out in the hills in a little hut. He is an example of how sensitive one can become through diet. Just for the experience, I tried the fruit diet and after a few weeks I felt very high and light. In my opinion, this fruitarian diet is just too fine for anyone working in the world.

Dr Swami Shankardevananda: This chart is a very useful aid to understanding diet. From what you say, it appears that most Indians would fit in somewhere between the yogis and the westerners. Their diet is much more naturally based; however, it is more processed than the yogic diet in that it is full of fats, fried food and milk products. Many Indians are also tending to adopt western habits, for example, they are eating more artificially flavoured, preserved and synthetic foods and much more meat. This is especially so in cities.

Dr Swami Vivekananda: It seems to me that the ashram diet is close to an ideal for most people. A little fruit, fresh garden vegetables, fresh legumes, brown rice and whole dairy products form a completely balanced diet. Vegetables should consist of a reasonable proportion of yellow and green, plus the cauliflower, cabbage, brussel sprouts and broccoli family. Yellow food, such as carrots, pumpkin, papaya and mangoes, contains carotene which is noted to be a very potent anti-cancer agent.

GEC Chicago carried out research on this project, involving thousands of men, which lasted probably more than 15 years. They concentrated on lung cancer, which is

Table 1: Degree of Processing

	Fresh or raw	Light cooking	Fried, fats	Frozen dried	Treated	Preserved, coloured	Synthetic
Fruit	from the tree			supermarket	packaged	jams, canned	jellies
Vegetable	from the garden			supermarket	packaged	canned	
Grain	organic, whole				polished white	precooked, packaged	
Nuts, Legumes	organic, whole						
Dairy	fresh milk	yoghurt	cottage cheese	dried milk	condensed milk	ice cream, cheese	
Meat	fish	chicken	pork		sausages	canned	
Junk	sweets etc.						

the commonest in the USA, and found a direct relationship between the amount of yellow food eaten and the non-incidence of cancer.

I advise people through this diagram that, if they are into all the heavy and heavily processed food, it is necessary to aim at changing the diet slowly to a more nourishing and less processed diet. We should understand that the quality of our nutrition depends on what we habitually eat. It is okay to have a bit of a treat now and then, but move back into the better diet on a regular basis.

Dr Swami Shankardevananda: It is not only the food itself; it is the way in which it is prepared. Garden vegetables which are fresh and full of goodness are spoiled by frying in a lot of oil.

Dr Swami Vivekananda: Frying destroys only certain nutrients. If you are vegetarian and eating green vegetables, you will be almost totally dependent on them for iron. People who are fresh fruit and raw vegetable eaters, for example, have a much higher incidence of pernicious anaemia and a very much higher incidence of iron deficiency. This is because the iron contained in the chlorophyll is not being released. You need to cook green vegetables before you can get the iron out.

Iron is mainly absorbed in the duodenum. If the food has not released its iron in a usable form before that point, it will pass out in the stool. You really need to cook green vegetables, preferably by boiling, not frying.

Dr Swami Shankardevananda: I have found that there are five main things to consider and these five points seem to be universal:

• Quantity of food
• Hunger
• Meal times
• Food combinations
• State of mind

Overeating is one of the biggest problems we face. Most people believe that dairy foods are good, and a certain

162

amount may indeed be necessary for a balanced diet, but if you take too much milk or too much of anything you get an imbalance.

Hunger is important because, if you are not hungry, any amount you eat is overeating. The time that you eat is important, of course, because your stomach's energy level and your capacity to digest food, has to be high. You will be overeating, for example, if you eat a heavy meal at 12 o'clock at night when your digestive energy is at its lowest point. Digestive energy is said to be highest between 9 and 11 a.m.

Combinations are important, for example, drinking milk with legumes, vegetables and grains, or after any meal, can create wind and constipation. A little bit of curd is okay, but too much creates problems.

State of mind is probably the most important. If we eat while we are worried, anxious, depressed or angry, for example, we not only do not feel hungry but our digestive juices are not properly secreted. A relaxed mind and good hunger is essential for good digestion.

Many people have digestive problems in India and in western countries which relate to overeating and excessive fats, spices and sugar in the diet. Food times are also incorrect. In India many people have tea in bed, breakfast at 9 o'clock, lunch at 2 o'clock, then tea and snacks at 6 o'clock and dinner at 10 o'clock. They hardly ever feel hungry and rarely fully enjoy what they eat. So I tell them to reverse their breakfast and meal times or, preferably, to cut out the evening snacks completely so that they have an early and light meal 3–4 hours before sleep so that digestion takes place. If they are hungry before sleep, they can have some fruit or a cup of tea (preferably with lemon).

Food is one of the biggest problems in terms of therapy. There is no doubt in my mind that we cannot tap healing energy unless we maintain a healthy manipura chakra through a light balanced diet.

Dr Swami Vivekananda: In the West more people have a better understanding of diet in terms of disease and they do not overeat so much as a rule. Of course, there are millions of people who eat an excess of fats and processed foods. Especially in the USA, and Australia to some extent, the food the average person is eating is really junk food, frozen food, television dinners and very highly processed things.

People ask me in the United States about diet supplements like vitamins and lecithin. Vitamin C has received a lot of publicity lately. Most of the vitamin C you get nowadays is synthetic, made from sugar. They just put an enzyme with it, forming ascorbic acid.

The principle behind the whole dietary question is that we require fuel. Cars and people run in the same way. Fuel is taken in and combined with oxygen to give off energy in the form of electrons plus certain wastes. In the human body the process gives off carbon dioxide and water, while in cars you get carbon monoxide, lead products and other noxious substances. However, when we are talking about diet, we have to go back to basics if we are to really get an understanding of what is going on.

Dr Swami Shankardevananda: The most basic food source of energy in the body is glucose which is stored in the liver as glycogen and in other tissues as fat. It is then mobilized and used whenever we need energy to fuel all the various processes in the body. Glucose is usually burned with oxygen (Krebs cycle) and eventually liberates energy, in the form of electrons, which is stored in phosphate molecules (adenosine triphosphate, ATP) to be liberated when required. One molecule of glucose gives a total of 36 ATP molecules, which is quite a lot of potential energy, plus carbon dioxide and water and other waste products, such as lactic acid.

Basically, in the body we have two main pathways for energy. The first is the one I just described, the Krebs cycle, also called substrate level phosphorylation, which stores energy for when it is required. The second pathway is the electron transport chain in which the energy stored in the phosphate molecule, the electron, is used to do some work such as building tissues, transportation, and so on.

Dr Swami Vivekananda: Sometimes the electrons produced by the metabolic processes are not used properly and they may attach themselves to the wrong place in the body. This means that energy is stored in the wrong place. Electrons attach themselves to different molecules giving those molecules an odd number of electrons. These electrons are very loosely attached to the molecules, and because these molecules travel throughout the body, the electron can easily jump off and attach itself to another part of the body, another molecule which is more attractive. This process damages the body. A chemical with an odd number of electrons is called a free radical.

In the normal healthy state we do not produce many free radicals and what we do produce is dealt with easily by a healthy body. However, when we are under stress, and who is not nowadays, or if we have lack of exercise, poor nutrition, constipation, illness, mental tension and anxiety, and so on, then we produce many more free radicals and the body is not fit to cope with them in its debilitated state. Free radicals are produced where the metabolism is overactive in relation to the body's need. There are certain areas in the body where electrons can cause tremendous damage and destruction and many researchers are convinced that this is causing the ageing process, cancer and many other diseases.

So this is one of the reasons why enough exercise, good nutrition, maintenance of good health and peace of mind are so important. Stress of any kind is a very important source of increasing the metabolism. Poor nutrition can be a source of stress, for example, substances which produce high bursts of energy, such as taking too much sugar, will overactivate the metabolism relative to body needs. This also highlights why yoga, as a method of regulating and balancing the metabolism by strengthening the body and relaxing the mind, is so important.

The three areas where damage can really take place are: the cell membrane, the immune system and the connective tissues.

1. Cell membrane: around every cell in the body is a membrane which usually has a fatty membrane around it. Stuck in the membrane are little blobs of protein, whose job it is to take food and other elements through the cell membrane to supply fuel, nutrients and various requirements to the cell. There are other proteins to take out the waste products and whatever else has to be carried out. It is thought that free radicals attach themselves to the fats and proteins in the cell membrane and change their structure and function so that the cell is rendered incapable of taking in and expelling materials efficiently. Even though there is plenty of food available in the body we cannot get it to where it is supposed to go.

In fact, many researchers now think that this is a major cause of diabetes. All the cell membranes in the body are affected by free radicals which render the cells less capable of taking in food from the bloodstream. This is thought to be a cause of the insulin resistance we see in advanced diabetes. These diabetics need vast amounts of insulin, not because the body is deficient in it (if you measure the blood insulin, it is high), but because the cells of the body are unable to take in glucose, which in turn is because the insulin cannot work properly on the cell membrane.

2. The immune system is the body's defence system. Along the capillaries of the different parts of the body that produce the immune substances are 'stem cells', which are like templates from which white blood cells are formed. One of these white blood cells is the so-called T-lymphocyte. These are the main cellular elements of the immune defence system which attach themselves to any bacteria, foreign material or cancer cell, which gets into the blood. These T-lymphocytes are then supposed to destroy the bacteria, cancer cell or foreign material.

If free radicals get into the stem cells and change the genetic constitution of these stem cells, then for the rest of that person's life that stem cell will always produce abnormal lymphocytes which are not effective. Then, over a long

166

period of time, say 50 to 70 years, the immune system becomes less and less effective as more and more of these stem cells become adversely affected by the free radicals.

Sometimes free radicals, it is thought, will change the genetic constitution so that the growth control mechanisms within the genes of the stem cells are so badly affected that the stem cells will grow without control. This is called leukaemia.

This same process can occur in any cell in the body. If a cell goes crazy it becomes a foreign substance to the body and it is the job of the lymphocytes and the antibodies to knock these cells out. In a normal person that is what occurs. In fact, we are probably producing cancer cells every day, but the lymphocytes and the immune defence system are supposed to monitor and destroy them. However, if these lymphocytes become inefficient due to free radicals attacking them, they are unable to do their job and cannot wipe out the malignant cells. This is thought to be one reason why people tend to get cancer, infectious conditions or many of the chronic illnesses.

The free radicals can, for example, also get into the joints of the body, especially affecting the cartilage and connective tissue, thereby changing their form. The body responds by producing antibodies from B-lymphocytes to these cells and this is what we call rheumatoid arthritis. This is one theory for auto-immune disease.

3. The connective tissues are also affected by free radicals and this produces the more visible processes of ageing such as hardening of the arteries, ligaments, joints, and so on. This is supposed to be due to cross linkage, where you have longitudinal connective tissue fibres in which free radicals have entered and due to their negative charge caused a misalignment and fusion of the fibres. This is what makes people look old. Wrinkles appear and creaking joints start seizing up. This process continues over a long period of time.

Dr Swami Shankardevananda: Actually, the free radical theory and yoga tie in together very well. Free radicals can be produced from stress and from disordering of our metabolic processes. Research from John Hopkins Institute at Baltimore, Maryland, states that excessive oxygen in the body can cause excess oxygen-free radicals (oxygen with an extra electron). For example, when someone has had a heart attack or heart surgery they are sometimes given extra oxygen to breathe and this extra oxygen has been found to combine with an electron to form a free radical which can cause havoc in the body.

So, even though we cannot survive without oxygen for more than a few minutes, too much oxygen acts like a poison. We also know that when we are under stress or tension or when we are very anxious, we tend to overbreathe, taking quick, shallow breaths. This is in order to feed the body's tissues, which are constantly demanding oxygen to cope with the stress; they are in a hypermetabolic situation. This is why stress causes the overproduction of oxygen free radicals, because we take extra oxygen into the body in order to cope with the stress. However, we are usually not utilizing the extra energy and oxygen through exercise, movement and activity. Most people just sit around and worry but they do not do anything positive about their problem. So, these unnecessary, useless oxygen molecules build up in the tissues because they are not metabolized and react to form free radicals which can then cause them damage.

Many people have said that the purpose of pranayama is to get more oxygen into the tissues. If this is so, then according to the above research this could be harmful. However, Swami Satyananda has always stated, and research into pranayama shows, that the purpose of pranayama and the majority of meditative pranayama techniques is to lead us into a relaxed, hypometabolic state, a meditative state in which the body and mind slow down and the demand for oxygen also slows. In this state the body needs less oxygen and we breathe more slowly. We can assume that whatever oxygen we take into the body is utilized fully and efficiently and no free radicals are formed. Research is needed on this point. Until it is done, however, we can say that pranayama and meditation, combined with a good lifestyle, would definitely be the best antidote for stress and free radicals and the most logical approach to a long and healthy life.

We know about the yoga side of things, how to do the practices and many of the effects, but how should we live and what should we eat in order to reduce the effects of stress?

Dr Swami Vivekananda: As the basic idea is to reduce the effects of stress and to decrease the number of free radicals being produced by the excess energy in the form of electrons, the first step is to produce only the energy and electrons we require and not have any left over to produce free radicals. Actually, electrons are required for all energy processes of the body. They are necessary for our metabolism, but if they are in excess, they are harmful. Therefore, as most people who are under stress do not get enough exercise, have poor nutrition, suffer from constipation and so on, they produce too many free radicals. This can be remedied, as you said, by the addition of yoga to our lives.

Reduction of stress, increase in exercise and good nutrition will prevent excess production of free radicals. Those extra free radicals which are produced will also be mopped up by the extra use of our muscles, which we get during asana, for example. A good diet also helps. There are certain substances in the diet called anti-oxidants (anti-free radical substances) which mop up free radicals. These are especially vitamins A, C and E, plus other vitamins and some minerals.

Vitamin A is found in carotene, the yellow pigment in pumpkin, carrots, corn, papaya and other orange vegetables and fruit. Carotene is two vitamin A molecules joined together, and when you take carotene into the body, it splits. For every molecule of that yellow pigment found in pumpkin, and so on, you get two vitamin A molecules. There is no question at all that in lung cancer, for example,

169

the increased incidence of the disease is proportional to the deficiency of vitamin A, carotene especially. It is fat soluble.

Vitamin C seems to be the most important antioxidant and electron 'mopper upper' for carbohydrate metabolism. Vitamin E seems to be the most important for fat metabolism. These vitamins, if taken in sufficient amounts, will check excess oxidation and free radical production. They mop up the extra electrons by a process of self-sacrifice, as it were, because these molecules are very attractive to the electrons.

Vitamin C, for example, is a carbohydrate and in some animals it is produced from the glucose in their bodies by their enzyme mechanisms. Gorillas produce 5000 mgs of vitamin C per day and adult gorillas average between two and two and a half times the size of an adult human being. This means that if we have anything like the metabolism of the gorilla – and in actual fact we presumably have much more stress and less exercise than gorillas do – that 2000–3000 mgs would probably be the limit of requirement for human beings per day. The allowance put forward by the Federal Drug Administration of the USA is only 65 mgs, which from this point of view seems to be too little.

One theory was put forward by one of the nutritionists who studied this (and a lot of really good in-depth medical research has been done) that a large percentage of the human race grew up in the tropics. In the tropics, fruit generally contains a much greater proportion of vitamin C. Any sort of fruit, for example oranges, if grown in the tropics, will have more vitamin C than those grown in cold climates. The average tree-ripened guava contains 1000 mgs of vitamin C, so two guavas fresh off the tree would probably supply the 2000 mgs of vitamin C for one day. However, as we increased in numbers and moved up into the cooler regions, we got into areas where there is a lower amount of vitamin C produced than in the tropics.

Dr Swami Shankardevananda: There is a theory that people who live in cold climates are more prone to developing antibodies and allergic reactions to citrus fruits, because in cold climates citrus fruits were not available until relatively recently. One researcher has developed a theory that the cause of arthritis is related to consumption of fruits which are not geographically locally grown.

Dr Swami Vivekananda: Vitamin E is found especially in yeast. A very high proportion of selenium is also found in yeast. These are also found in the germ of grains and to some extent in soya beans. These are the main sources. Vitamin E is also found in fat, and this is one of the main ways it is taken in. It is found in dairy fats, for instance, only however if the animals have sufficient vitamin E in their own diet, but now of course many animals are being fed on highly refined foods. They are given pellets that are supposed to contain everything, but there is uncertainty about their real nutritional value.

It is said that for humans 400 units of vitamin E and probably about 25–50 mg of selenium are required every day. The theory is that to slow down the disease and ageing process, people need to eat the required amounts of these vitamins and minerals. However, when you are taking gas-ripened fruit, highly processed and canned foods, etc., it is difficult to know how much vitamin C you are taking, so in this situation we probably need a multivitamin supplement.

Just by taking a piece of fruit off a tree, the vitamin C content starts dropping. It is also immediately destroyed by boiling water. If you look at grains of the highly polished and refined rice most people eat, the germ, the little space where the vitamin E was, is no longer there. Only whole grains have it. Cracked brown rice or wheat, for example, is good. I think Indians generally make up their vitamin requirements from the whole wheat they use in chappatis, even though they eat white rice. The people in south India, who mainly eat rice and not rotis, are in an area where the fruit contains a very high amount of vitamin C anyway.

Dr Swami Shankardevananda: Certain foods are high in these vitamins and we should probably eat more of these on

171

a regular basis. Cauliflower, broccoli, brussel sprouts, carrots and citrus fruits contain high amounts of vitamins A, C and E.

The food thought to contain the most carcinogens, cancer-causing agents, are charred foods. Apparently the heating of amino acids causes this. Burnt toast and charcoal broiled steaks would be the worst offenders. Of course, there are the fatty foods, salt-cured and smoked foods, artificially coloured and flavoured foods, synthetic foods, chemically treated foods and pesticides and other chemicals which find there way into food and are known to be cancer causing. Hatha yoga shatkarmas, asana and pranayama, combined with a healthy diet, will help us to eliminate these poisons from our body.

An obvious question that arises out of all of this is where does ashram food fit in? We eat very little fruit and no milk. Of course, this diet has a spiritual purpose and is designed to maintain brahmacharya, but where do we get our B12 and C vitamins from?

Dr Swami Vivekananda: All the greens have some vitamin B12 and adults don't need that much. When you get older you tend to need more. Vitamin B12 is stored, and a meal with a fair amount of B12 could be stored for six months, but if you are on just a fruit diet, you are not getting any B12 at all. On a fruit and fresh greens diet, it is very unlikely that you would take in any B12 at all, and it needs to be available in the stomach to bind with the intrinsic factor which allows it to be absorbed.

It looks as though you can get along on low amounts of vitamin C. However, if people take a high amount of vitamin C over a period of time and then reduce this intake so that they take in the amount in an ordinary diet, which has approximately 60–70 mg and which kept them going well previously, then these people would actually develop the symptoms of scurvy for some time. So, somehow the mechanisms become dependent on that high amount of vitamin C. Now if people stay a long time on a low amount of vitamin C, maybe their systems adapt to that too.

Dr Swami Shankardevananda: Many vitamins such as C are synthesized in animals, either by enzymes or with the help of bacteria. Even in human beings, bacteria produce vitamin K, B12, thiamine, riboflavin and other substances in the large intestine. However, these cannot be absorbed. We have to take in these vitamins nutritionally, via food. We have a varied diet while most animals eat either a vegetarian diet as herbivores, or meat as carnivores. Few animals are omnivores like humans, eating both meat and vegetables and such a large variety at that.

It may be that humans originally manufactured their own vitamins inside their own body but as they started to eat certain foods the internal production decreased. We see this phenomenon even today; for example, when we give someone cortisone in tablet form, the manufacture of cortisone in the body decreases by a negative feedback mechanism. If this occurs over a long time, we may lose the capacity to synthesize cortisone and become dependent on an external source. So, perhaps this also occurred with vitamins. As humans began to cultivate external sources of vitamins, the body did not need to produce its own. Of course, we still produce our vitamins D and K in the body, but sufficient vitamins A, the B group, C and E must be taken in regularly.

I believe that, if we sustain a vegetarian diet minus vitamin C input, the body has the capacity to create its own vitamin C, though it may take time. I am sure we can eventually evolve this capacity if it is necessary. It may be possible to do this in one lifetime if we use yoga practices, especially the hatha yoga shatkarmas and meditation in combination with asana and pranayama.

There would probably have to be a transition diet between the old and new states in which yoga purifies, relaxes and strengthens, and this would probably be minus fruit and milk products. I suspect that the eventual outcome of such a diet would be a higher state of consciousness, a totally new way of seeing the world; there would be a definite correlation between gross and higher conscious states.

Of course, such a state would be difficult to achieve, and a long way off for most people. Many of the great saints and yogis probably enter into states of altered body metabolism as they enter higher states of consciousness and their diet changes appropriately. During their sadhana they may eat only chappati, dal and a little vegetable, or only fruit and milk, though I believe the former is more common especially amongst sadhus in the Himalayas.

Probably the most important thing for most people living in the world, practising a gentle sadhana program, is to take a light, balanced diet of grains, pulses, vegetables, fruits, and a little milk from time to time. The most important thing to avoid is excess fats and oily, greasy and fried foods. Excess of these foods might also interfere with vitamin C absorption because they would coat the intestines with fat.

Dr Swami Vivekananda: It is known that the excessive intake of non-digestible fats like mineral oil, paraffin oil, etc. can produce deficiencies of fat soluble vitamins A, D, E, but I don't see this interfering with water soluble vitamin C.

Dr Swami Shankardevananda: Yes, by leaching it out. If you have excessive consumption of fat or oil, you do not have the liver capacity to dissolve fat. The liver produces bile, which is like a soap, to dissolve fat. If we get fat on our hands, we need soap or we cannot get the fat off our hands. So you have this excess, undigested fat in your intestines, which prevents not just water soluble vitamins from being absorbed, but many other things as well. This may be one of the reasons why laghoo shankhaprakshalana works so well, by cleaning out all the rubbish which prevents us digesting and absorbing all the valuable nutrients we need so much for our health and vitality.

So we should have a light diet which is relatively low in fat. If you look at the diet of the Hunzas and other long-lived people, you will see that they have a very low fat intake. That is one of the highlights of their diet. It is very similar to an ashram diet, which is mainly carbohydrate – 60% of calorie intake, maybe 400–500 gms of carbohydrate, 50–100

174

gms of protein, 10–20 gms of fat per day – these are the main constituents of the ashram diet, and this is sufficient to maintain a healthy, active body.

Dr Swami Vivekananda: One thing we should also consider is that when people come into the ashram they sometimes feel sick with this diet.

Dr Swami Shankardevananda: The reason for this is that people come into an ashram after being on a poor diet and their bodies and minds are in a very impure and dissipated state. They have a lot more problems disease-wise in the initial adjustment phase. People who have had a heavy diet before they come here may get covered in ulcers and sores if the process of purification is too fast.

Dr Swami Vivekananda: What they should do is slowly come off the meat diet before they go on to a pure vegetarian diet. Maybe all those people who have been on a vegetarian diet for many years are in fact producing the herbivorous, vitamin C producing enzymes or bacteria in their intestines, and the meat eaters are not. That is very interesting.

Dr Swami Shankardevananda: What about vitamin B? We know we are getting plenty of it in wheat and it is very important in neurological functions. Also what about vitamin D?

Dr Swami Vivekananda: Vitamin D is especially important for children's brain formation. Children should really have milk but there is no necessity for adults to drink milk, even people on a vegetarian diet, because there is calcium in the vegetables, if they eat enough.

Dr Swami Shankardevananda: What about the other minerals like selenium and magnesium? There is so much research into these areas now.

Dr Swami Vivekananda: For people under a lot of stress and tension, who find it difficult to balance their food intake, for example, eating at odd times and in different places due to work or social commitments, I recommend they take 1000–2000 mgs of vitamin C per day. Vitamin E and selenium are usually contained in a good multivitamin preparation.

I look at this as a necessary evil for people with irregular meals and unavoidable stress in their daily lives. They are all producing free radicals due to stress and irregular food habits. So, along with the yoga, they most probably need to add extra vitamins A, C and E, either in the form of food or as a vitamin supplement.

Dr Swami Shankardevananda: Actually, we know very little about diet from the scientific point of view. For years scientists have been saying that we need first class protein in the form of meat, fish, eggs, and so on, and that vegetarian diets were unable to fulfil these needs, then they realized that a vegetarian diet is sufficient. One thing is certain, that a vegetarian diet is conducive to a longer lifespan and less risk of cancer of the large intestine. We see vegetarian groups such as the Seventh Day Adventists living several years longer on average than a comparable group of non-Adventists.

A study reported in the February 1984 *Science Digest* on the latest research from researchers Paul Sagall and Paola Timiras at the University of California, Berkeley, shows that a diet deficient in tryptophan, the essential amino acid for growth, more than doubled the lifespan of some mice from 701 days to 1527 days and increased their reproductive life from 15 to 33 months. That is the equivalent of an 80-year-old woman giving birth. Of course, these rats were stunted and sick in many ways and many died of the deficiency.

However, the study shows us that we still have a lot to learn about what we eat. It may be that a high protein intake, especially too much meat, is responsible for a lot of disease, degeneration and early ageing. Once again we see the yogic maxim working; balance is essential.

The most important dietary regulation is to eat in moderation, and only what you can digest. This food restriction principle was first seen at Cornell University in the 1920s and has been repeatedly confirmed. Animals who eat less from an early age live anywhere from 25–100% longer.

At UCLA, Roy Walford and Richard Woindruch have taken fish, which usually live only one year, and extended their lifespan to three years by reducing diet and water temperature. Both fasting and a cool environment reduce metabolism which probably reduces free radicals and therefore does not wear out the body as quickly as a higher metabolism. We can understand this if we think that a candle with a large flame will burn out faster than one with a small flame.

Space scientists also believe that one of the effects of living in space will be to extend the lifespan. When we live without gravity we need less food, fuel and energy because there is no more walking, lifting or heavy exertion. Therefore, we eat less, lower our metabolism and live longer.

The best and most practical way for us to lower our metabolism is to eat less and make the diet light, low in fats and fried food. At the same time, occasional fasting and regular meditation practice will lower the metabolic rate and should help us to live longer, fight stress more effectively, think clearly and intuitively, and generally live a better life. This formula will help us no matter when we start to implement it, though research clearly shows that the earlier we start the better it is.

Summing up, the ideal diet for increased longevity is the ashram diet. People who are long-lived, perhaps up to the age of 135 years or more, live in the Hunza Valley, in the Hindu Kush in Pakistan, the Caucasus Mountains in Georgia and the Villcabamba Valley in the Andes of Ecuador. Apart from living in a clean, pure mountain environment and leading an active life, they are said to eat only 1800–2000 calories per day, half as much as most people in affluent countries. Their diet is remarkably like ashram food except that they eat fruits and some dairy products.

What it all boils down to is to eat a light, simple and balanced diet, low in fat and sugar and high in fruits, sprouted mung or other pulses and plenty of clear liquids and water.

177

Dr Swami Vivekananda: I advise people in the West to move away from highly processed foods and a poor nutritive diet, and to keep slowly moving up the healthy diet ladder. It is not good doing this too quickly or fanatically, rather they should go as slowly as they like, but never reach the pure food trip because it is just too fine for most people.

Practical Digestion

22

Path to Good Health

Before we can do anything practical to treat digestive disorders, we must first locate the cause, whether in the body or mind. Once this has been found, we can select and follow the correct path, that which is easiest and most direct, to the destination of good health. Indigestion, in most cases, is caused by factors as anxiety, tension, frustration, guilt, resentment, and so on. Be sure, however, that in your case it is not an organic thing, and that there is nothing physically wrong which may require medical treatment.

The body is a whole organism and depends on each organ functioning in balance with all the other organs for its continued good health. When a basic process such as digestion is out of order the whole organism is affected. To prevent minor digestive problems from snowballing into other major disorders, we suggest that you start examining your lifestyle and habits now. Try to weed out all destructive habits and plant health-giving ones in their place. In doing this, some important points to remember are:

1. Be aware of your eating habits and your mind while taking food.
2. Do not worry about the future. The catastrophes you anticipate rarely occur.
3. Be aware of those situations which cause the most stress and try to resolve them. It is impossible not to be affected

by the expectations of others, but try not to let them control your life.

Digestive disorders, as a whole, are very easy to treat by using yoga. Start now and you will be sure of good health in the near future. With regularity and determination, it is remarkable how much can be achieved in a short time. However, it is no good just talking about doing something or sitting around reading a book. You must act now. If you delay, you will regret your apathy later.

Advice and precautions

The root cause of indigestion can be reached and resolved through yoga, and the likelihood of recurrence is negligible if you continue the practices. It should be remembered that each individual is different and requires specific techniques to suit his/her own particular needs. Therefore, an experienced, qualified teacher is essential, especially when therapy is sought. The teacher acts as an objective observer who can see from experience just what you need. With expert guidance you are certain to make good progress. Here are a few helpful suggestions for those who wish to start on the yogic path to good health:

- Never go to extremes and practise more than you are capable of. Yogic techniques are designed to remove tension, but you must relax while doing them. Never exert undue effort or strain; the attitude should be effortless, relaxed concentration.
- The stomach should be empty before commencing the practices. After eating allow four to five hours to elapse, depending on whether you have taken a big or small meal.
- While practising, always breathe through the nose unless instructed to do otherwise.
- Practise on a folded blanket laid on a clean floor.
- If possible designate a well ventilated room where there is peace and quiet for your practices. The room should not have a draught or objects cluttered around that may distract the mind or impede bodily movement.

The yogic practices and general improvements in your lifestyle may require a major change in schedule and habits. It might well be difficult in the beginning, but don't worry and don't get discouraged if at first you do not succeed. Overcoming old conditioning is always a test of our desire for self-improvement. Once you have made the change and find yourself becoming healthier, your entire attitude to life will change. Long after your digestive upsets are a thing of the past, you will continue to grow, becoming physically and emotionally healthier than you dreamt possible.

Note: Full details of all the recommended practices can be found in *Asana Pranayama Mudra Bandha* by Swami Satyananda Saraswati, published by Yoga Publications Trust. However, all techniques should be learnt under personal instruction from an experienced teacher. For further guidance in finding a qualified teacher please contact the Bihar School of Yoga, Munger 811201, Bihar, India, or visit the website: www.biharyoga.net.

23

Daytime Sadhana

Many people think yogic practices are limited to the early hours of the morning and so they fail to appreciate the broader view of sadhana. Spiritual practice is not an end in itself, but a means to achieve harmony within the body and mind. We move through the process of sadhana into a heightened perception of the world and begin to see with clarity and precision the things we previously missed completely. With the yogic eye, a broad new expanse opens before us, and we are able to see the whole life process as one evolving continuum.

Sadhana gives many benefits throughout the day. It makes us feel much lighter, stronger and more capable of functioning in the world. No matter where we are or what we are doing, we generally experience the yogic attitude of awareness accompanied by greater control and peace of mind. This increases our enjoyment of every activity and gradually we begin to understand that every position of the body is an asana, every breath a pranayama, every gesture a mudra and every thought and feeling a part of a meditative process.

Simple daily activities such as eating and defecation can also become extensions of our morning practice. We can experiment in order to determine what effect awareness has on eating, or meditation on digestion and defecation. With practice we can utilize the basics of sadhana to improve and

184

enhance our life from moment to moment. Once we accustom ourselves to yoga we find innumerable occasions to apply it and thereby improve all aspects of our lives.

While eating

Before eating: Before you start to eat ensure that you are fully relaxed and that your sympathetic nervous system is dominant. Your right nostril should be flowing and if it is not then perform padadhirasana (the breath balancing pose) for a short time.

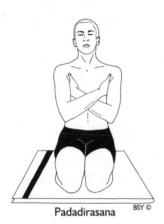

Padadirasana   BSY ©

Sit in vajrasana and cross the arms in front of the chest, placing the hands under the armpits with the thumbs pointing upward in front of you. Close your eyes and become aware of the breath in the nostrils. Your breath should be slow and rhythmical. If the left nostril is open and the right closed, remove the left hand and continue with just the right hand in the left armpit. This should open the right nostril automatically after a few minutes of practice.

During a meal: When commencing your meal become aware of your body, breath and mind. Relax each and every part. You may imagine that you are eating with your favourite deity, God, guru or the higher self. The best sitting position during the meal is sukhasana (the easy pose).

It is good for young and old alike as it does not require very much flexibility of the knee joints. It is better than sitting on a chair because crossing the legs moves the prana up from the lower part of the body and pelvis into the abdomen, making more energy available for the digestive organs.

During the meal ensure that your breath is slow, smooth and relaxed. Your awareness should be on your food fully,

185

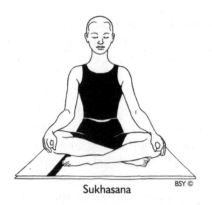

Sukhasana

both before it enters the mouth and also afterwards. In this way you can appreciate the sensation of each mouthful of food mixing with the saliva in your mouth as you chew and then travelling down the oesophagus to the stomach. Each taste, the temperature and texture of the food should be thoroughly experienced. When you finish the meal you should be aware of the food that has passed down into your stomach and the digestive process which is already underway. This is the meditation of eating.

Always try to end each meal as soon as your stomach is filled to satisfaction. If you continue beyond this point it is possible to eat and eat, but without satisfaction, stretching the stomach until a feeling of bloated overfullness is reached. For many people this is the starting point of indigestion. Eating beyond this point dulls the mind and decreases energy as it overworks the digestive system.

After eating: After meals you should sit in vajrasana (thunderbolt pose). In the beginning you can maintain the posture for as long as is comfortable. Slowly build up the time to 20 minutes. While sitting you will notice that even though you may have been able to eat more, your hunger is satisfied and you still feel light.

Try to become aware of your digestive tract. Visualize your digestive tract. Visualize it inside your abdomen and become fully aware of all of its movements, sensations or

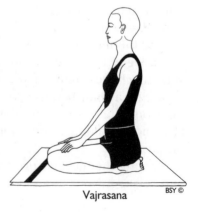

Vajrasana

186

feelings. Use your knowledge of anatomy and physiology of the digestive tract to visualize ideal digestion in progress in you body.

Alternatively, you can just focus on the rhythmical movement of the natural breath in the abdomen. The more you relax with awareness, the better your digestion will be. You can also count each respiration from 108 back to 1 or from 54 to 1. Should you lose count, then go back to the starting number. If feelings, visions and thoughts bubble up spontaneously, simply observe them with the detached attitude of a silent observer, and return your awareness to the breath.

Another variation is to visualize a sun with its centre at the navel, radiating power throughout the whole of the body. Feel its warmth digesting the food and sending prana and nutrients to all the different parts of the body.

On the toilet

Toilet training for children is a matter of common sense and trial and error. For many of us who have had an ineffective and also inhibition-producing toilet training and are now suffering the consequences, awareness and a few simple yogic practices can undo all the damage and set us back on the path of good health.

The best sitting position to use for defecation is the squatting position. This position helps the natural energies function and indeed is the most ideal for people suffering from constipation. This was the natural position assumed for defecation before sitting-type toilet arrangements became fashionable. Now, unfortunately, many people have lost the ability to squat. In order to better approximate the natural optimal posture, they tend to lean forward, crowding the eliminatory organs and constricting the energies.

In order to relearn squatting the best asanas are the pawanmuktasana part 3 (shakti bandha) series which include: nauka sanchalanasana (rowing the boat), chakki chalanasana (churning the mill), rajju karshanasana (pulling the rope),

187

kashtha takshanasana (chopping wood), namaskarasana (salutation pose), vayu nishkasana (wind releasing pose) and udarakarshanasana (abdominal stretch pose). Though at first you may feel a little uncomfortable, mentally and physically, you will quickly appreciate the efficacy of this position once you have become accustomed to it. Squatting helps us to relieve not only constipation and piles, but also other pelvic conditions such as premenstrual tension as well as reducing fat on the hips and aiding the flow of pelvic energies.

The next time you are on the toilet, whether squatting or sitting, watch your body and mind as in the process of antar mouna. Examine the toilet habits you have developed over your lifetime and observe the thoughts, actions, reactions and feelings you experience. Try to be a witness of your natural body mechanisms so that you are aware of each and every occurrence from start to finish. Internal awareness induces relaxation and parasympathetic activity. Chin mudra helps to gain inner awareness and to channel the spinal energies into the abdomen.

Become aware of the natural breath in the abdomen. Feel the rhythmic inward and outward movement and just let whatever is going to happen, happen. Do not strain. Accept the situation as it is, even if no stool is expelled.

Imagine that you are breathing through the spinal cord. With every inhalation the breath ascends the spinal cord and with every exhalation it descends the spinal cord. You are ascending from mooladhara to ajna and descending from ajna to mooladhara. Repeat this for a few minutes using ujjayi pranayama. When you are established in this breath awareness, visualize the intestines, especially the large intestine, which travels up the right side of the abdomen, from right to left across the upper abdomen, and down the left side of the abdomen. After some time you should begin to actually feel and become aware of the movement of faeces and gas.

As you inhale take the breath up the spinal cord to ajna and as you exhale bring the breath down to manipura chakra at the navel area and feel the exhaled prana filling the whole abdomen. The more you exhale, the more relaxed your abdomen becomes and the more movement you can feel and actually visualize within the colon. Repeat this for some time.

Then, while maintaining the inhalation to ajna and exhalation to manipura, slowly expand the abdominal muscles slightly and keep them rigid but relaxed. Do not strain. You should feel a slight increase in the intra-abdominal pressure. The abdomen still moves with the breath but it is controlled. Feel as though you are holding the internal organs mentally and squeezing faeces out of the rectum.

Under stress and strain

Whenever you feel too much tension, there are a few simple techniques which can be employed to relax the body and mind. Probably the best of these is yoga nidra or shavasana with breath awareness. Even if you are unable to lie down during the day, you can still utilize basic breath awareness anytime, anywhere – in the car, bus or train, on the job or while eating, walking or talking. All that is necessary for this practice is awareness of your breath, preferably in the abdomen. Feel the rhythmic movement and keep the breath as relaxed, slow and natural as possible. Feel yourself actually riding the breath. With every exhalation you breathe out impurities and toxins, worries, tensions, problems and frustrations. With every inhalation you breathe in warm, golden, life-giving energy. Feel more and more relaxed and refreshed with every breath.

This should be practised as often as possible during the day. Try to extend it into all your daily activities. In the beginning you may use a special reminder to trigger your memory. For example, every time you look at a clock or watch, practise this for at least five minutes.

Another variation of this practice is to use the pulse as a counting measure. Take hold of the left hand pulse with the right hand. When you feel the pulse, count five beats for each inhalation and five for each exhalation, or whatever number of beats you feel comfortable with. Within a few breaths you will notice the pulse slowing and the breathing becoming longer and deeper. Continue for as long as you have time.

With practice, yogic techniques can be adapted to suit all the needs of daily life. In terms of alleviating chronic tension and indigestion, these and other techniques should be combined with karma, bhakti and jnana yogas. This integral approach is a powerful means of changing the consciousness and eliminating the causes of disharmony and disease on all levels.

24

Relaxing the Abdomen

Tension at the emotional, mental or spiritual levels of our being is reflected in the body as muscle tension. This can be easily demonstrated – when we become mentally tense, we tighten our muscles. The main areas of tension are found in the neck, jaw and abdomen. Of course, all muscle groups tighten, but some are easier to relax consciously than others. The abdominal muscles are perhaps the easiest muscle group to relax.

The following two practices are simple, effective and practical. They require very little time and effort and are very helpful in the prevention and cure of digestive disorders.

Tadagi mudra

Tadagi mudra (barrelled abdomen technique) is a simple practice which relaxes the abdomen.

Technique

Sit with the legs outstretched and grasp the big toes with both hands. Inhale as deeply as is comfortable so that the chest and abdomen are fully expanded.

Then retain the breath for a few moments and focus your awareness on the abdominal muscles, which are pushed forward as far as possible.

Exhale and relax the abdomen.

Tadagi may be repeated up to 10 times.

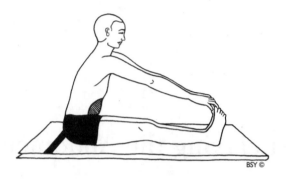

Benefits: After finishing this practice you will feel a relaxation of tension in the abdominal region. Tadagi mudra offers the perfect counter to tense, tightly constricted abdominal musculature. By pushing the abdomen out and simultaneously filling the lungs with air, we increase the pressure inside the abdominal cavity. This stimulates and tones the abdominal nerve plexuses and organs, and enhances lymphatic drainage. Manipura chakra, which governs the digestive fire, is also stimulated. When the abdomen relaxes, all the other muscle groups of the body are similarly affected because of the central effects on the brain.

Manipura shuddhi

We lose power in manipura chakra because of tension and anxiety. At the physical level, tension reflects as poor solar plexus and adrenal gland function, resulting in the symptoms of indigestion. One of the best methods of dealing with this tension is manipura shuddhi, which is preferably practised in any comfortable meditation posture.

Technique

Breathing in ujjayi pranayama, inhale through the navel and straight back to manipura chakra, located in the spinal cord.

Retain the breath and awareness at manipura and mentally repeat the bija (seed) mantra *Ram* three times.

192

Then exhale, moving the breath plus awareness forward and out of the navel.

Be aware of the breath moving in and out of the navel centre and the rhythmic expansion and contraction of the abdomen. Concentration is not required in this practice, only awareness.

25

Hatha Yoga

Hatha yoga is concerned with purification of the physical body. In its traditional form there are six cleansing practices, which are called the hatha yoga *shatkarmas*, or cleansing techniques. They are:

1. *Neti*: cleaning the nasal passages. There are two main forms:
   i) jala neti performed with warm saline water
   ii) sutra neti performed with a catheter.
2. *Dhauti*: washing the alimentary canal from the mouth to the anus. There are 5 main forms:
   i) *Danta dhauti* is cleaning of the teeth. There are other dhautis for the tongue, eyes, ears and scalp
   ii) *Vatsara dhauti* is cleaning the stomach with air, also called bhujangini mudra
   iii) *Varisara dhauti* or *shankhaprakshalana*, in its long and short form, is washing the entire alimentary canal with warm saline water
   iv) *Vahnisara dhauti* or *agnisar kriya* is the rapid expansion and contraction of the abdomen
   v) *Hrida dhauti* is purification of the chest using a stick (danda dhauti), a cloth (vastra dhauti) and by vomiting (vaman, or kunjal, and vyaghra kriyas).
3. *Nauli*: churning of the abdominal wall to massage and strengthen the abdominal organs.
4. *Basti*: washing of the large intestine by taking water through the anus.

5. *Kapalbhati*: purification of the frontal brain by air and water.
6. *Trataka*: the practice of steady gazing.

Of the six hatha yoga cleansing techniques, only dhauti, basti and nauli are of particular importance in the direct treatment of digestive disorders. We will deal first with dhauti as its range of application and usage is wide and most beneficial.

Note: These shatkarmas should be learned from and practised under the guidance of an experienced yoga teacher in a therapeutic setting. For complete details of the practices consult the book *Asana Pranayama Mudra Bandha*, published by Yoga Publications Trust.

Kunjal Kriya or Vaman Dhauti (the practice of vomiting water)

Probably the most practical and easy to perform of the dhautis is kunjal kriya (the practice of vomiting water). It has a multiplicity of variations and can be used in almost all types of indigestive processes, especially acidity and gas, nausea, food poisoning and auto-poisoning, and dyspepsia. Kunjal is undoubtedly the most widely used cleansing practice and its assimilation by medical practitioners will be of practical benefit to many people suffering not only from digestive disorders but also asthma, headache, epilepsy, and so on.

Technique

Kunjal is performed by drinking tepid, saline water up to the point where you feel like vomiting.

The water should be lukewarm and contain one teaspoon of salt per litre (more salt can be added if necessary). Drink at least six glasses in quick succession, and if you can, continue drinking right up to the point where it is not possible to swallow even one sip more.

At this point you may vomit automatically. If not, then put two fingers down your throat and massage the back of the tongue as far down as possible. By pressing it you will feel the urge to vomit and water will come up in a series of quick gushes.

Continue pressing until the stomach is empty.

Precautions: After kunjal wait for at least 20 minutes before eating food.

Time of practice: Kunjal should be done first thing in the morning and followed by neti. It is also done after shankhaprakshalana.

Contra-indications: Kunjal should not be performed by people suffering from hernia, high blood pressure, raised intracranial pressure, heart disease, stroke, acute peptic ulcer, or by diabetics with eye problems.

It should be learned and performed under guidance in a therapeutic setting.

Practice note: Kunjal has none of the unpleasant sensations usually associated with vomiting, like nausea and bad smell. The water brought up is usually clean and without bad odour. Because of added salt, mucus and dirt are dissolved and the acid is diluted. The water contains nothing solid so it comes out quickly and easily, making you feel light, fresh and clean inside.

Vyaghra Kriya (tiger practice)

Vyaghra kriya is the ideal technique for digestive upsets such as chronic dyspepsia or heartburn when there is excessive stomach acid, as well as when there is insufficient gastric secretion. It differs from kunjal in that it is classically performed three hours after taking a meal rather than on an empty stomach. However, it can occasionally be practised immediately after eating if there is heaviness or discomfort in the stomach, or if the food is felt to have been contaminated or to be in any way harmful. Vyaghra is a natural method and like many yogic practices it was copied directly from animals. The tiger gorges itself on its prey and then regurgitates the remnants of the food from the stomach three or four hours later. Dogs and cats use this technique whenever they have eaten something which does not agree with them. They eat grass as an emetic and then vomit out the gastric contents, ridding themselves of the poisons that have entered their system.

Technique

Perform three hours after eating, if there is still heaviness, discomfort, belching or bringing up of contents from the stomach.

Follow exactly the same procedure as for kunjal but repeat the practice two or three times until only clean water comes up.

While performing vyaghra kriya try to keep food particles from entering the nose.

It is advisable to do neti straight afterwards so as to clean the whole nasal passage in case irritating fluids have entered.

By removing the burden of indigestible foods, vyaghra restores energy, lightness and well-being.

Practice note: Vyaghra kriya should be done only when necessary. The same restrictions apply as for kunjal.

Shankhaprakshalana or Varisara Dhauti (washing of the intestines)

In yogic therapy no course for indigestion is complete without shankhaprakshalana (washing of the intestines). The most complete and powerful of yogic cleansers, this technique can accomplish in a few hours what may take days or weeks by ordinary fasting. Its effects, although profound at a physical level, are even more intense at the pranic and mental levels.

This practice has two forms: a long course which can be performed once or twice a year under supervision and which takes about two hours to complete, and a short course (laghoo) which can be performed every morning, if necessary, in about 10 to 15 minutes.

Shankhaprakshalana cleans the entire digestive tract and frees any old and dried refuse that has become stuck to the walls of the intestines over a period of years. At the same time it allows the digestive system a chance to rest, perhaps for the first time in years. Rebalance occurs in the whole of the digestive tract, including secretion of acids and alkalis, juices, enzymes, proteins and so on. Laghoo shankhaprakshalana (short intestinal wash) has the same effect, slowly dislodging impacted particles and dirt which have been clogging the mucous membranes and preventing secretion and absorption of nutrients.

The dietary restrictions after the practice also help rebalance the digestive system. The cleansing process that has been initiated by the salt water continues during this time in much the same way as a fast, with elimination proceeding faster than absorption.

After shankhaprakshalana you feel very light, and many report a definite alteration of consciousness. This is because the combination of water travelling down the digestive tract and the various asanas stimulate chakras in the spinal cord. This releases a lot of unconscious mental constipation as well as physical constipation. By cleaning the body we also clean the mind, and there is actually a change in the level of our awareness, for by this practice we are altering the state of our cellular consciousness. Shankhaprakshalana is highly recommended for sufferers of constipation, gas, acidity, indigestion and for many other disease conditions when performed under expert guidance.

Technique
Preparation: Shankhaprakshalana should only be performed under expert guidance in a happy and relaxed atmosphere.

The best time is at the beginning of the spring or when the weather is good and the mind is relaxed.

It is practised on an empty stomach and involves drinking at least 16 or more glasses or warm saline water.

In preparing saline water it is important to remember that the first six glasses should be hotter with a little more salt, while the remaining glasses should be warm with the minimal amount of salt necessary for the practice.

Complete intestinal wash: Drink two glasses of salty water as quickly as you can. Then perform the following 5 asanas 8 times each: tadasana, tiryaka tadasana, kati chakrasana, tiryaka bhujangasana and udarakarshanasana (these asanas are fully described in chapters 26 and 28). These asanas help to relax the sphincters of the digestive tract and allow the water to pass freely and quickly to the anus for discharge.

Drink two more glasses of salty water and repeat all 5 asanas again 8 times each.

Drink two more glasses and perform the 5 asanas 8 times each a third time.

After the third time, go to the toilet and try to evacuate the bowels.

Relax. Do not strain.

After a minute or so in the toilet, come out and drink two more glasses.

Continue this process: drink two glasses of salty water then do the asanas 8 times each. Go to the toilet. Eventually some kind of motion will occur.

At first solid stool will start to be evacuated and then water and stool mixed. Carry on drinking water, doing the 5 asanas and sitting on the toilet.

Eventually the water that you pass will be clean. On an average, between 16 and 20 glasses of salty water must be consumed before clean water is evacuated. Some people will take less and some will take more.

It is important to stop the practice when the water becomes almost clear as the system may start producing bile indicated by bright yellow water.

Immediately after completing shankhaprakshalana perform kunjal and neti to complete the cleansing process and also to raise the energies.

Rest: Total rest is essential after completing shankhaprakshalana. Lie down or sit quietly for exactly 45 minutes, keeping the body warm. It is important that you do not sleep. During this period of time the whole digestive system is being completely rested and revitalized.

Special food: Khichari, a preparation of rice and dal (lentils) cooked together with ghee (clarified butter) must be eaten 45 minutes after shankhaprakshalana. This is necessary to activate and lubricate the digestive tract in a gentle manner.

Further rest: After eating, further rest is necessary for the remainder of the day. Do not sleep for three hours after the first meal. Take only khichari for the next meal six hours later.

Frequency: People with normal health can perform shankhaprakshalana twice a year with great benefits. It should be performed in an ashram environment for best effects.

Food restrictions: These are necessary for at least one week after shankhaprakshalana. Chemically processed, non-vegetarian and acidic food should be strictly avoided. Milk, buttermilk and acidic fruits such as lemons, grapefruit and oranges are also restricted. Alcohol, cigarettes, tea, coffee and betel nut preparations such as pan are forbidden. For one week the diet should be pure, simple and as non-acidic as possible. After cleaning the whole digestive tract, a sudden introduction of toxic or difficult to digest food might produce bad reactions such as fever, indigestion, constipation and all those things you are trying to rid yourself of.

Contra-indications: People suffering from any medical condition should seek guidance from a qualified yoga teacher before attempting shankhaprakshalana, especially those taking medication. This practice should also be avoided during pregnancy. Those with chronic amoebic dysentery, active ulcers, high blood pressure, heart disease or in a weakened condition should not attempt this practice.

Laghoo Shankhaprakshalana (short intestinal wash)

This is the shorter version of the full practice of shankha-prakshalana. It is perhaps the most effective yogic technique for removing chronic constipation. The effects are not quite as dramatic as the full version, but because it can be performed every day the effects accumulate and result in a slow but progressive increase in energy, purity of body and mind and overall health.

Technique

Perform first thing in the morning on an empty stomach. Prepare water in the same way as described for shankha-prakshalana.

Drink two glasses of salty water and then practice the same 5 asanas 8 times each. Repeat this twice more.

After six glasses of water you should go to the toilet. Usually there is a clear bowel movement plus a large quantity of urine.

Frequency: For therapeutic purposes, it may be practised daily for a limited period of time under expert supervision. Otherwise practising once or twice a week is sufficient. On completion of the practice rest for half an hour before taking food or drink.

Contra-indications: As for shankhaprakshalana.

Jala Neti (nasal cleansing with water)

Neti is used to clear the nasal passages after kunjal, vyaghra kriya and shankhaprakshalana. For this practice a *neti lota* (small pot with a long spout) is used to pour warm salt water through the nostrils.

Technique

Fill the neti pot with warm water mixed with salt in the ratio of one teaspoonful per half litre.

Tilt the head to the right and gently insert the spout in the left nostril so that the water flows through the nasal cavity and out the right nostril.

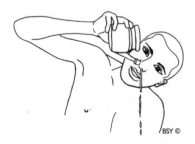

Repeat the process on the other side.

After completing this process the nostrils must be thoroughly dried.

Close the right nostril with the right thumb and breathe in and out quickly through the left nostril 10 times as in kapalbhati pranayama. Do not blow too hard.

Repeat through the right nostril.

Perform once more through both nostrils.

Contra-indications: This practice should not be done by people with chronic bleeding in the nose without expert advice.

Vastra Dhauti (cloth cleansing)

This practice is especially good for acidity, wind and poor digestion. It is a more difficult practice, however, and should not be attempted without expert guidance. It should only be performed on a completely empty stomach.

Technique

A special cloth of fine cotton or gauze, approximately 2½ cms wide and 3 metres long is used to clean the throat, chest and stomach. The cloth is soaked in warm water until it is soft.

Place one end of the cloth in the mouth.

Moisten it well with saliva in the mouth before swallowing. Carefully and slowly swallow it in the same way as you would food.

Drink a little water every minute or so to make the cloth go down more easily.

202

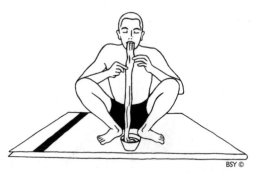

Don't swallow all the cloth. Hold one end loose so that it can eventually be withdrawn.

Keep the cloth in the stomach no longer than 20 minutes or it will begin to pass through the intestines.

Advanced practitioners may perform nauli or agnisar kriya.

Do not speak while practising.

After completing vastra dhauti, kunjal can be performed to wash out what the cloth has loosened from the stomach wall.

Then do neti to complete the cleaning process.

Contra-indications: This practice should not be performed by people suffering from hypertension, heart disease or stroke, during illness, when the body is weak, or until two or three months after surgery.

Agnisar Kriya or Vahnisara Dhauti (activating the digestive fire)

Agnisar kriya removes gas and constipation, tones up all the digestive organs and stimulates the appetite. It is should be practised on an empty stomach.

Preparatory practice: Swana Pranayama (panting breath)

Sit in vajrasana and separate the knees as far as possible. Breathe in deeply. Exhale, emptying the lungs as much as possible.

Place both hands on the knees and lean forward slightly, keeping the arms straight.

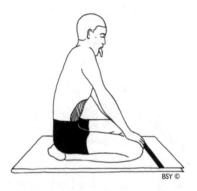

Open the mouth and extend the tongue.

Breathe in and out while simultaneously expanding and contracting the abdomen. The breathing should resemble the panting of a dog.

Do not strain.

Breathe in and out 10 to 20 times.

This is one round.

In the advanced form (Agnisar Kriya) the action is performed with external breath retention.

Contra-indications: People suffering from high blood pressure, heart disease, acute duodenal or peptic ulcers, overactive thyroid gland or chronic diarrhoea should not perform this kriya.

Nauli (abdominal massaging)

In this practice, churning of the rectus abdomini, the two long muscles running down the centre of the abdomen, massages all the abdominal organs and the digestive tract. Thus it is a powerful method of removing all digestive ailments, particularly constipation, nervous diarrhoea, acidity and wind. However, it is a difficult practice and takes time to perfect. It should not be attempted until uddiyana bandha and agnisar kriya have been perfected. Both should be practised in the cooler months.

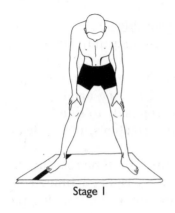

Stage 1

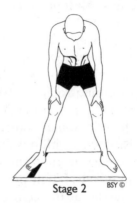

Stage 2

BSY ©

Technique
Stage 1: Madhyama nauli (central abdominal contraction)

Stand with the feet a metre apart.

Place the hands on the thighs and bend the knees slightly.
Perform jalandhara bandha while maintaining external
breath retention.

Contract the rectus abdomini muscles so that they form
a central arch running vertically in front of the abdomen.
Hold for as long as is comfortable.

Release and return to the upright position. Inhale deeply
allowing the abdomen to expand.

Relax the whole body.

This is one round.

Relax in the upright position until the heartbeat returns
to normal.

This stage should be perfected before proceeding to the
next stage.

Stage 2: Vama nauli (left isolation)

Isolate the rectus abdomini muscles at the left side of the
abdomen.

Stage 3: Dakshina nauli (right isolation)

Isolate the rectus abdomini muscles at the right side of
the abdomen.

Proceed to stage 4 only after perfecting this practice.

Stage 4: Abdominal rotation or churning
This practice should not be attempted until stages 1–3 have been mastered.

Practise vama nauli, then rotate the muscles to the right, dakshina nauli, and back to the left, vama nauli.

Continue rotating the muscles from side to side.

Start by practising 3 consecutive rotations, then release the abdominal contraction.

Next start with dakshina nauli first, this time rotating the muscles from right to left, left to right, 3 times consecutively. Then perform madhyama nauli, isolating the muscles at the centre.

Raise the head and return to the upright position.

Inhale slowly and deeply, allowing the abdomen to expand. This is one round.

Duration: Start with 5 rounds of stage 1 and work up to 10. Stages 2 and 3 should be performed together, 5 to 10 rounds each.

Precautions: Nauli should only be practised under expert guidance. If pain is felt in the abdomen during nauli, stop the practice immediately.

Contra-indications: Nauli should not be attempted by people suffering from heart disease, hypertension, high blood pressure, hernia, gallstones, acute peptic ulcers, or those recovering from internal or abdominal surgery.

Pregnant women should not practise nauli.

Basti (yogic enema)
This is the yogic enema which cleans the colon and removes gas. It is useful for constipation, piles, dysentery and chronic diarrhoea. This practice is not recommended for daily use; once or twice a week is enough.

Technique
Basti is ideally performed standing in a flowing river.

Lean forward and place the hands on the knees.

Draw water into the bowel by expanding the anal sphincter

muscles and performing uddiyana bandha and nauli.
Hold the water in the bowels for some time, then expel it
through the anus.

Precaution: This technique should be learned under expert
guidance.

Moola Shodhana (anal cleansing)

Moola shodhana purifies the anus and rectum and is
excellent for removing piles. In the *Gherand Samhita* (1:43–
45) it says: "If a person does not practise moola shodhana,
then the apana does not pass freely. Clean the anus with a
soft turmeric plant or with the finger. Then repeatedly wash
it with water. This practice removes the hard, fermented
stool from the lower colon. Abdominal ailments are removed,
the body becomes graceful and healthy and one's digestive
fire improves."

The turmeric root is medicinal and has antiseptic
properties. It stimulates the nerves of the anus and rectum
and helps to encourage peristalsis and a free flow of blood to
the area. If turmeric is not available, the third finger is just
as effective and can be used as a substitute.

Technique

This technique is performed in a squatting position.

First lubricate the turmeric root or your third finger with
water, vaseline or ghee and then insert it as far into the
rectum as it will go.

Rotate the root or the finger around the inner surface of
the anal sphincter 10 times clockwise and then 10 times
counter-clockwise.

The practice can be intensified by performing ashwini
mudra with the root of the finger inside the anus.

Wash the area intermittently and repeat until the anus
and rectum are clean.

It is good to perform this technique before basti.

26

Pawanmuktasana Series

This set of asanas is especially designed for those people who have not practised yoga before and whose bodies are too stiff to attempt the major asanas immediately. Though they seem relatively simple, if practised correctly they are a very powerful means of relaxing, coordinating and synthesizing the brain, mind and digestive process.

PART 1: ANTI RHEUMATIC GROUP

These asanas loosen up the joints of the body. They are performed sitting in the base position:

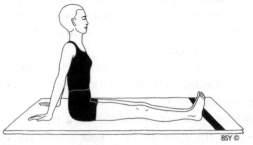

Base position
Sit with the legs outstretched, feet slightly apart. Place the palms on the floor just behind the buttocks. Lean back slightly, using the arms to support the back. Close the eyes and relax the whole body in this position.

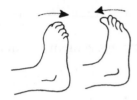 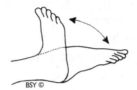

Padanguli Naman (toe bending)

Move the toes of both feet slowly backward and forward. Hold each position for a few seconds.

Repeat 10 times.

Breathing: Inhale as the toes move backward. Exhale as the toes move forward.

Goolf Naman (ankle bending)

Keep the feet slightly apart. Slowly move both feet backward and forward, bending them from the ankle joints. Hold each position for a few seconds.

Repeat 10 times.

Breathing: Inhale as the feet move backward. Exhale as the feet move forward.

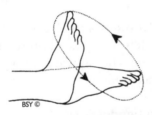

Goolf Chakra (ankle rotation)

Separate the legs a little, keeping them straight. Keep the heels on the ground throughout the practice.

Stage 1: Slowly rotate the right foot clockwise from the ankle 10 times and then repeat 10 times anti-clockwise. Repeat with the left foot.

Stage 2: Place the feet together. Slowly rotate both feet together in the same direction. Do not allow the knees to move.

Practise 10 times clockwise and then 10 times anti-clockwise.

Breathing: Inhale on the upward movement. Exhale on the downward movement.

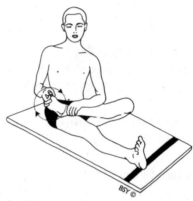

Goolf Ghoornan (ankle crank)
Bend the right knee and place the foot on the left thigh.
Hold the right ankle with the right hand and the toes of the right foot with the left hand.
With the left hand, slowly rotate the right foot 10 times clockwise.
Then practice 10 times anti-clockwise.
Repeat with the left foot placed on the right thigh.
Breathing: Inhale on the upward movement.Exhale on the downward movement.

Janu Naman (knee bending)
Bend the right knee and clasp the hands under the right thigh.
Straighten the right leg, pulling up the kneecap.
Keep the hands under the thigh but straighten the arms.
Do not allow the heel or toes to touch the floor.
Bend the right leg at the knee so that the thigh comes close to the chest and the heel near the right buttock.
This is one round.

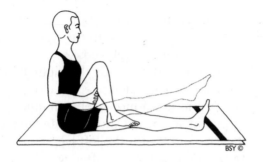

Practise 10 rounds with the right leg and then with the left leg.

Breathing: Inhale while straightening the leg. Exhale while bending the leg.

Ardha Titali Asana (half butterfly)

Bend the right leg and place the right foot as far up on the left thigh as possible.

Place the right hand on top of the bent right knee and hold the toes of the right foot with the left hand.

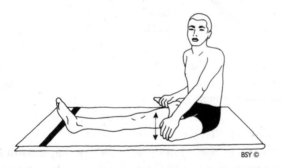

Stage 1: With breath synchronization

While inhaling, gently move the right knee up towards the chest. Exhaling, gently push the knee down towards the floor.

The leg muscles should be passive, the movement being achieved by the exertion of the right arm.

Slowly practise 10 up and down movements.

Stage 2: Without breath synchronization

Remain in the same position with the right leg on the left thigh and the leg muscles relaxed.

Push the right knee down with the right hand towards floor and release, letting the knee move back by itself.

Practise 30 up and down movements in quick succession. Breathing should be normal and unrelated to the practice. Repeat stages 1 and 2 with the left leg.

Practice note: To unlock the leg after completing stage 2, bring the bent knee in front of the chest, then slowly and carefully straighten the leg.

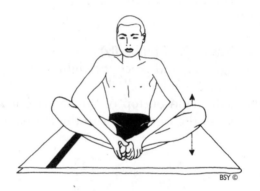

Poorna Titali Asana (full butterfly)

Bend the knees and bring the soles of the feet together, keeping the heels as close to the body as possible.

Fully relax the inner thigh muscles.

Stage 1: Clasp the feet with both hands.

Gently bounce both knees up and down, pushing the knees towards the ground on the downward stroke.

If the legs are stiff use the elbows as levers to press the legs down.

Practise 30 to 50 up and down movements.

Stage 2: Keep the soles of the feet together.

Place the hands on the knees. Using the palms, gently push the knees down towards the floor, allowing them to move up again.

Do not force this movement.
Repeat 20 to 30 times.
Straighten the legs and relax.

Breathing: Breathe normally.

Contra-indications: People with sciatica and sacral conditions
should avoid this asana.

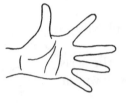 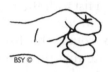

Mushtika Bandhana (hand clenching)

Hold both arms straight in front of the body at shoulder
level. Open the hands, palms down, and stretch the
fingers as wide apart as possible.

Slowly close the fingers with the thumbs inside to make a
tight fist.

Again open the hands and stretch the fingers.

Repeat 10 times.

Breathing: Inhale on opening the hands. Exhale on closing
the hands.

Manibandha Naman (wrist bending)

Stretch the arms in front of the body at
shoulder level.

Keep the elbows straight, the palms open
and fingers straight throughout the
practice.

Bend the hands backward from the
wrists as if pressing the palms against a
wall with the fingers pointing toward
the ceiling.

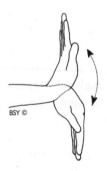

Bend the hands forward from the wrists
so that the fingers point toward the
floor.

Bend the hands up again for the next round.

Repeat 10 times.

Breathing: Inhale with the backward movement. Exhale with the forward movement.

Manibandha Chakra (wrist joint rotation)

Stage 1: Extend the right arm forward at shoulder level.

Make a fist with the right hand, with the thumb inside.

Slowly rotate the fist about the wrist, ensuring that the palm faces downward throughout the rotation.

The arms and elbows should remain perfectly straight and still.

Practise 10 times clockwise and 10 times anti-clockwise.

Repeat with the left fist.

Stage 2: Extend both arms in front of the body with the fists clenched. Rotate both fists together in the same direction. Practise 10 times in each direction.

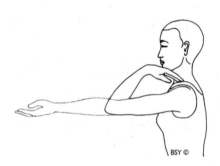

Kehuni Naman (elbow bending)

Stage 1: Stretch the arms in front of the body at shoulder level. The hands should be open with the palms facing up.

Bend the arms at the elbows and touch the fingers to the shoulders. Straighten the arms again. This is one round. Repeat 10 times.

Stage 2: Extend the arms sideways at shoulder level, hands open and palms up.

Bend the arms at the elbows and touch the fingers to the shoulders. Again straighten the arms sideways.

Repeat 10 times.

Breathing: Inhale while straightening the arms. Exhale while bending the arms.

Practice note: The upper arms remain parallel to the floor, elbows at shoulder level.

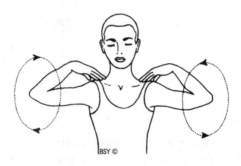

Skandha Chakra (shoulder socket rotation)

Stage 1: Place the fingers of the right hand on the right shoulder.

Rotate the right elbow in a large circle.

Practise 10 times lowering the elbow first and then up to 10 times raising the elbow.

Repeat with the left elbow.

Stage 2: Place the fingers of the left hand on the left shoulder and the fingers of the right hand on the right shoulder.

Fully rotate both elbows at the same time in a large circle. Practise 10 times lowering the elbows first and then 10 times raising the elbows.

Breathing: Inhale on the upward stroke. Exhale on the downward stroke.

215

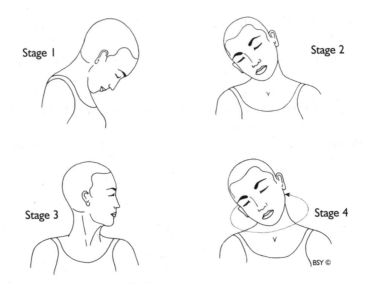

Stage 1

Stage 2

Stage 3

Stage 4

BSY ©

Greeva Sanchalana (neck movements)

Stage 1: Close the eyes. Slowly move the head forward and try to touch the chin to the chest.

Then move the head as far back as is comfortable.

Do not strain.

Practise up to 10 times.

Breathing: Inhale on the backward movement. Exhale on the forward movement.

Stage 2: Slowly move the head to the right bringing the right ear towards the right shoulder without turning the head or raising the shoulders.

Move the head to the left side bringing the left ear towards the left shoulder.

This is one round. Practise up to 10 rounds.

Breathing: Inhale on the upward movement. Exhale on the downward movement.

Stage 3: Keep the head upright and the eyes closed.

Gently turn the head to the right so that the chin stays in line with the shoulder. Slowly turn the head to the left as far as is comfortable. Keep the chin at the same level from the floor throughout. Do not strain.

Practise up to 10 times on each side.

Breathing: Inhale while turning to the front. Exhale while turning to the side.

Stage 4: Remain in the same position with the eyes closed. Slowly rotate the head, first downward, then to the right, backward and then to the left side in a relaxed, smooth, rhythmic, circular movement.

Practise up to 10 times clockwise and then up to 10 times anti-clockwise. Do not strain.

After the practice, keep the neck straight and the eyes closed.

Breathing: Inhale as the head moves up. Exhale as the head moves down.

Contra-indications: Stage 4 should not be performed by elderly people and those suffering from low blood pressure, very high blood pressure or cervical spondylosis.

PART 2: DIGESTIVE/ABDOMINAL GROUP

These asanas strengthen the digestive system and eliminate energy blockages in the abdominal area.

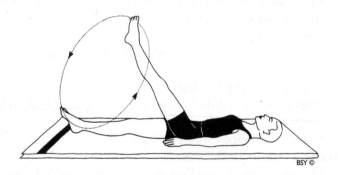

Chakra Padasana (leg rotation)

Lie flat on the back.

Raise the right leg 5 cm from the ground, keeping the knee straight.

Rotate the entire leg clockwise 10 times in as large a circle as possible.

The heel should not touch the floor at any time during the rotation.

Rotate 10 times in the opposite direction.

Repeat with the left leg.

Do not strain. Rest until the respiration returns to normal.

Breathing: Breathe normally throughout the practice.

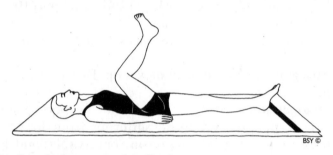

Pada Sanchalanasana (cycling)

Stage 1: Lie flat on the back.

Bend the right knee and bring the thigh to the chest.

Raise and straighten the leg completely.

Then, lower the straight leg in a forward movement.

Bend the knee and bring it back to the chest to complete the cycling movement.

The heel should not touch the floor during the movement.

Repeat 10 times in a forward direction and then 10 times in reverse.

Repeat with the left leg.

Breathing: Inhale while bending the knee and bringing the thigh to the chest.

Exhale while lowering the leg.

Stage 2: Raise both legs.

Practise alternate cycling movements as though peddling a bicycle.

Practise 3 to 5 times forward and then 3 to 5 times backward.

Breathing: Breathe normally throughout.

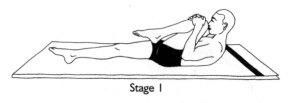

Stage 1

Stage 2

BSY ©

Supta Pawanmuktasana (leg lock pose)
Stage 1: Lie flat on the back.
  Bend the right knee and bring the thigh to the chest.
  Interlock the fingers and clasp the hands just below the right knee.
  Keep the left leg straight and on the ground.
  Inhale deeply, then while exhaling raise the head and shoulders off the ground and try to touch the right knee with the nose. Hold the breath out in the final position for a few seconds, counting mentally.
  While slowly inhaling, return to the base position.
  Relax the body.
  Repeat 3 times with the right leg and then 3 times with the left leg.
Stage 2: Bend both knees and bring the thighs to the chest.
  Interlock the fingers and clasp the hands just below the knees.
  Practise the same movement as in stage 1 but with both legs together, 3 times.
Contra-indications: Those suffering from high blood pressure or serious back conditions, such as sciatica or slipped disc, should not perform this practice.

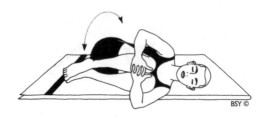

Jhulana Lurhakanasana (rocking and rolling)

Stage 1: Lie flat on the back. Bend both legs to the chest. Interlock the fingers and clasp the hands just below the knees.

Roll the body from side to side 5 to 10 times, touching the sides of the legs to the floor.

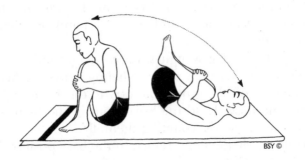

Stage 2: Squat with the buttocks just above the floor.

Rock the whole body backwards and forwards on the spine.

Try to come into the squatting position on the feet when rocking forward.

Practise 5 to 10 backward and forward movements.

Breathing: Breathe normally throughout.

Contra-indications: Not to be performed by persons with serious back conditions.

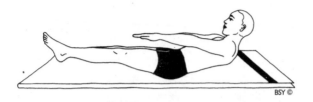

Naukasana (boat pose)

Lie flat on the back, palms down. Keep the eyes open throughout.

Breathe in deeply. Hold the breath and then raise the legs, arms, shoulders, head and trunk off the ground.

The shoulders and feet should be no more than 15 cm off the floor.

The arms should be held at the same level and in line with the toes.

Remain in the final position and hold the breath.

Breathe out and return to the supine position. Relax the whole body.

This is one round. Practise 3 to 5 rounds.

Relax in shavasana after each round.

Variation: Repeat the same process as above but tense the whole body in the raised position.

Contra-indications: Not to be performed by persons with high blood pressure.

PART 3: SHAKTI BANDHAS

These asanas improve the energy flow within the body.

Gatyatmak Meru Vakrasana (dynamic spinal twist)

Sit with the legs outstretched.

Separate the legs as far apart as is comfortable.

Stretch the arms sideways at shoulder level.

Keeping the arms straight, twist to the left and bring the right hand down towards the left big toe.

Stretch the left arm behind the back, keeping both arms in a straight line.

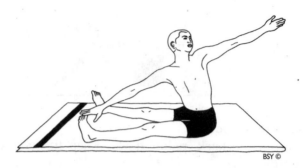

Turn the head to the left and gaze at the left hand.

Twist in the opposite direction and bring the left hand down towards the right big toe.

Stretch the right arm behind the back. Turn the head to the right and gaze at the right hand.

This is one round.

Practise 10 to 20 rounds.

Breathing: To apply pressure in the abdomen: breathe in when twisting and breathe out when returning to the centre.

Contra-indications: People with back conditions should avoid this asana.

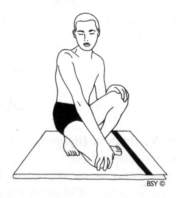

Kawa Chalasana (crow walking)

Squat on the floor with the feet apart and the buttocks above the heels.

Place the palms of the hands on the knees.

Begin to take small steps in the squatting position. Walk either on the toes or the soles of the feet.

Practise up to 50 steps and then relax in shavasana.

Breathing: Breathe normally throughout.

Contra-indications: People suffering from disorders of the knees, ankles or toes should not practise this asana.

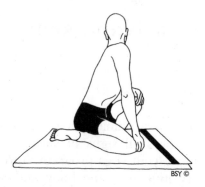

Udarakarshanasana (abdominal stretch pose)

Squat with the feet apart and the hands on the knees.

Breathe in deeply. Breathe out, bringing the right knee near to the left foot.

Push the left knee towards the right, simultaneously twisting to the left.

Keep the inside of the right foot on the floor.

Try to squeeze the lower abdomen with the combined pressure of both thighs.

Look over the left shoulder.

Hold the breath out for 3 to 5 seconds in the final position.

Breathe in when returning to the starting position.

Repeat on the other side of the body to complete one round.

Practise 5 rounds.

Note: *This is one of the asanas for shankhaprakshalana.*

27

Surya Namaskara

The practice of surya namaskara revitalizes the whole body and removes all signs of sleep, making it an excellent way to begin your yoga program. It loosens all the joints, flexes every muscle in the body and activates the respiratory and circulatory systems. Regular practice regulates the flow of prana in ida and pingala nadis, leading to a balanced energy system at both physical and mental levels. Its benefits are innumerable.

Surya namaskara consists of twelve physical postures that correspond to the signs of the zodiac. Each position is associated either with inhalation, or retention, or exhalation, so that the whole sequence is synchronized with breathing. This breath flow must not be forced or unnatural. Awareness is as essential in surya namaskara as in all yogic practice. Without awareness most of the potential of this practice is lost. On completion of the practice, relaxation is essential to allow the body to return to normal. Shavasana with constant awareness of the breath is the most recommended procedure.

Sequence for learning
One should first familiarize oneself with the twelve positions and for some time be concerned only with mastering the physical movements. Once you find that you can perform all the movements automatically, with little conscious

direction, then synchronize the breath with the movement. Awareness should then be on both breath and movement.

Tempo and number of rounds: At first surya namaskara should be performed slowly to ensure correct development of the movement and breathing. However, with regular practice your body will flow smoothly through the positions and you will be able to perform them faster. You may then speed up the practice, but always ensure that the breath does not become shallow. The number of rounds depends on individual health and time available. Surya namaskara should never be practised to exhaustion.

Preparation: Surya namaskara should always be practised on an empty stomach. Before commencing, stand with the feet together or slightly apart and arms hanging loosely by the side of the body. Close the eyes gently and become aware of the whole physical body. Relax the body mentally.

Note: For further information on this practice refer to *Surya Namaskara: A Technique of Solar Revitalization*, published by Yoga Publications Trust.

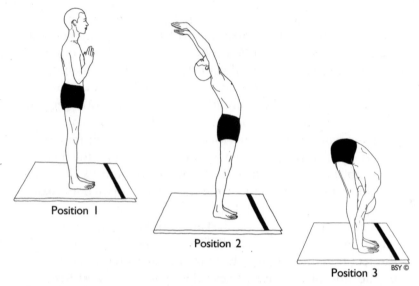

Position 1

Position 2

Position 3   BSY ©

Position 1: Pranamasana (prayer pose)

Remain standing upright with the feet together.

Place the palms together in front of the chest in namaskara mudra.

Relax the whole body.

Breathing: Breathe normally.

Position 2: Hasta Utthanasana (raised arms pose)

Raise and stretch both arms above the head, separating the hands shoulder width apart.

Bend the head, arms and upper trunk backward slightly.

Breathing: Inhale while raising the arms.

Position 3: Padahastasana (hand to foot pose)

Bend forward until the fingers or palms of the hands touch the floor on either side of the feet.

Try to touch the knees with the forehead.

Do not strain.

Keep the knees straight.

Breathing: Exhale while bending forward.

Contra-indications: People with back conditions should not bend forward fully. Bend only as far as comfortable.

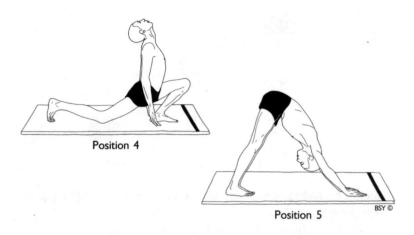

Position 4

Position 5

BSY ©

Position 4: Ashwa Sanchalanasana (equestrian pose)

Place the palms of the hands flat on the floor beside the feet.

Stretch the right leg back as far as possible.

At the same time, bend the left knee, keeping the left foot on the floor in the same position. Keep the arms straight. In the final position, the weight of the body should be supported on both hands, the left foot, right knee and toes of the right foot. The head should be tilted backward and the back arched.

Breathing: Inhale while stretching the right leg back.

Position 5: Parvatasana (mountain pose)

Take the left foot back beside the right foot.

Simultaneously, raise the buttocks and lower the head between the arms, so that the back and legs form two sides of a triangle.

The legs and arms should be straight in the final position.

Try to keep the heels on the floor in the final pose.

Do not strain.

Breathing: Exhale while taking the left leg back.

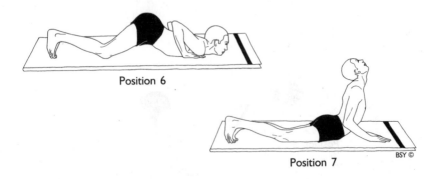

Position 6

Position 7

BSY ©

Position 6: Ashtanga Namaskara (salute with eight parts or points)

Lower the knees, chest and chin to the floor.

In the final position only the toes, knees, chest, hands and chin touch the floor.

The knees, chest and chin should touch the floor simultaneously. If this is not possible, first lower the knees, then chest, and finally the chin. Buttocks, hips and abdomen should be raised.

Breathing: Hold the breath outside.

Position 7: Bhujangasana (cobra pose)

Lower the buttocks and hips to the floor.

Straightening the elbows, arch the back and push the chest forward into the cobra pose. Bend the head back.

The thighs and hips remain on the floor and the arms support the trunk. Unless the spine is very flexible the arms will remain slightly bent.

Breathing: Inhale while raising the torso and arching the back.

Position 8: Parvatasana (mountain pose)

· This stage is a repeat of position 5.

From bhujangasana assume parvatasana.

The hands and feet do not move from position 7.

Raise the buttocks and lower the heels to the floor.

Breathing: Exhale while raising the buttocks.

Position 9: Ashwa Sanchalanasana (equestrian pose)

This stage is the same as position 4.

Keep the palms flat on the floor.

Bend the left leg and bring the left foot forward between the hands. Simultaneously, lower the right knee so that it touches the floor and push the pelvis forward.

Tilt the head backward.

Breathing: Inhale while assuming the pose.

Position 10: Padahastasana (hand to foot pose)

This position is a repeat of position 3.

Bring the right foot forward next to the left foot.

Straighten both knees.

Bring the forehead as close to the knees as possible without straining.

Breathing: Exhale while performing the movement.

Position 11: Hasta Utthanasana (raised arms pose)

This stage is a repeat of position 2.

Raise the torso and stretch the arms above the head.

Keep the arms separated shoulder width apart.

Bend the head, arms and upper trunk backward slightly.

Breathing: Inhale while straightening the body.

Position 12: Pranamasana (prayer pose)

This is the final position and is the same as position 1.

Bring the palms together in front of the chest.

Breathing: Exhale while assuming the final position.

Positions 13–24: The twelve positions of surya namaskara are practised twice to complete one round. Positions 1 to 12 constitute half a round. In the second half, the positions are repeated with two small changes:

i) In position 16, instead of stretching the right foot backward, stretch the left foot back.

ii) In position 21, bend the right leg and bring the right foot between the hands.

Conclusion: On the completion of each half round, lower the arms to the side, relax the body and concentrate on the breath until it returns to normal. After completing surya namaskara, practise shavasana for a few minutes.

Duration: Beginners should start with 2 or 3 rounds and add one more round every few weeks to a maximum of 12 rounds.

Contra-indications: The practice of surya namaskara should be immediately discontinued if fever, acute inflammation, boils or rashes occur. These may develop due to excess toxins in the body. When the toxins have been eliminated, the practice may be resumed.

Surya namaskara should not be practised by people suffering from high blood pressure, coronary artery diseases, or those who have had a stroke. It should also be avoided in cases of hernia or intestinal tuberculosis.

People with back conditions should consult a medical expert before commencing this practice.

During the onset of menstruation, this practice should be avoided.

28

Major Asanas

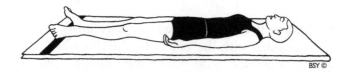

Shavasana (corpse pose)

Lie flat on the back with the arms about 15 cm away from the body, palms facing upward.

A thin pillow or folded cloth may be placed behind the head to prevent discomfort.

Let the fingers curl up slightly.

Move the feet slightly apart to a comfortable position and close the eyes.

The head and spine should be in a straight line.

Make sure the head does not fall to one side or the other.

Relax the whole body and stop all physical movement.

Become aware of the natural breath and allow it to become rhythmic and relaxed.

Duration: According to time available. In general, the longer the better although a minute or two is sufficient between asana practices.

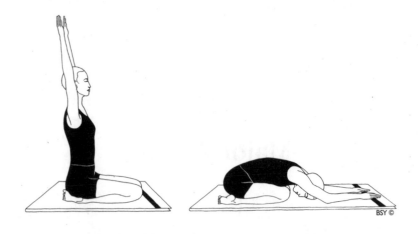

Shashankasana (pose of the moon or hare pose)

Sit in vajrasana with the palms on the thighs.

Inhaling, raise the arms above the head, keeping them straight and shoulder width apart.

Exhale while bending the trunk forward from the hips, keeping the arms and head in line with the trunk.

At the end of the movement, the hands and forehead should rest on the floor.

Retain the breath out for up to 5 seconds in the final position.

Then, simultaneously inhale and slowly raise the arms and trunk to the vertical position.

Breathe out while lowering the arms to the knees.

This is one round.

Practise 3 to 5 rounds.

Duration: Beginners should slowly increase the length of time in the final position after the last round until they are able to hold it comfortably for at least 3 minutes.

Contra-indications: Not to be performed by people with very high blood pressure, slipped disc or those who suffer from vertigo.

Tadasana (palm tree pose)

Stand with the feet together or about 10 cm apart, and the arms by the sides.

Raise the arms over the head, interlock the fingers, turning the palms upward, and place the hands on top of the head.

Keep the eyes fixed on a point on the wall slightly above eye level.

Inhale and stretch the arms, shoulders and chest upward.

Raise the heels coming up onto the toes. Stretch the whole body, holding the breath and the position for a few seconds.

Lower the heels while breathing out and bring the hands back to the top of the head.

This is one round.

Practise 5 to 10 rounds.

Breathing: Synchronize the breath with the raising and lowering of the arms.

Variation: Tadasana may also be performed while gazing up at the interlocked fingers.

Note: *This is one of the asanas for shankhaprakshalana.*

Tiryaka Tadasana (swaying palm tree pose)

Stand with the feet about 2 feet apart. Fix the gaze on a point in front.

Interlock the fingers and turn the palms outward.

Inhale and raise the arms over the head.

While exhaling, bend to the left side from the waist.

Do not bend forward or backward or twist the trunk.

Hold the position for a few seconds while retaining the breath outside. Inhale and slowly come to the upright position. Repeat on the right side.

233

From the upright position exhale while bringing the arms down to the sides. This completes one round.

Practise 5 to 10 rounds.

Variation: The fingers may be interlocked with the palms facing downward.

Note: *This is one of the asanas for shankhaprakshalana.*

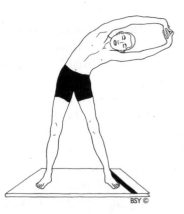

Kati Chakrasana (waist rotating pose)

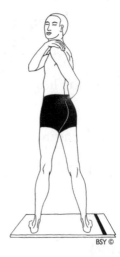

Stand with the feet about half a metre apart and the arms by the sides.

Take a deep breath in while raising the arms to shoulder level. Breathe out and twist the body to the left.

Bring the right hand to the left shoulder and wrap the left arm around the back to the right side of the waist. Look over the left shoulder as far as possible, keeping the back of the neck straight and head upright.

Hold the breath for two seconds and accentuate the twist.

Inhale and return to the starting position.

Repeat on the other side to complete one round.

Keep the feet firmly on the ground while twisting.

Practise 5 to 10 rounds.

Practice note: This asana may be performed in a more dynamic way by swinging rhythmically with the arms without synchronizing the movements with the breath.

Note: *This is one of the asanas for shankhaprakshalana.*

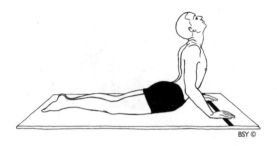

Bhujangasana (cobra pose)

Lie flat on the stomach with the legs straight and feet together, and the forehead on the floor.

Place the palms of the hands flat on the floor under the shoulders.

Slowly raise the head, neck and shoulders, then using the back muscles start to raise the trunk.

Then begin using the arm muscles and raise the trunk further, straightening the elbows to raise the trunk as high as possible and arch the back. Gently tilt the head backward.

In the final position, the pubic bone remains in contact with the floor.

Hold the final position.

To return to the starting position, slowly bring the head forward, release the upper back by bending the arms and lower the navel, chest, shoulders and finally the forehead to the floor.

This is one round.

Breathing: Inhale while raising the torso.

Breathe normally in the final position or retain the breath if the pose is held for a short time.

Exhale while lowering the torso.

Duration: Practise up to 5 rounds, gradually increasing the length of time in the final position.

Contra-indications: People suffering from peptic ulcer, hernia, intestinal tuberculosis or hyperthyroidism should not practise this asana without expert guidance.

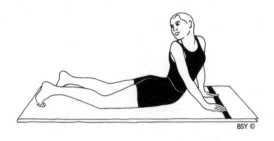

Tiryaka Bhujangasana (twisting cobra pose)

Assume the final position of bhujangasana with the legs separated about half a metre.

The toes should be tucked under and the heels raised, so that the foot rests on the ball of the foot.

The head should be facing forward.

Twist the head and upper portion of the trunk and look over the left shoulder.

Gaze at the heel of the right foot.

In the final position, the arms remain straight or slightly bent as the shoulders and trunk are twisted.

Try to feel a diagonal stretch of the abdomen.

Relax the back and keep the navel as close to the floor as possible.

Stay in the final position for a few seconds.

Face forward again and repeat the twist on the other side without lowering the trunk.

Return to the centre and lower the body to the floor.

This is one round.

Breathing: Inhale while raising.

Retain the breath inside while twisting to both sides.

Exhale while lowering to the floor.

Duration: Practise 3 to 5 rounds.

Note: *This is one of the asanas for shankhaprakshalana.*

236

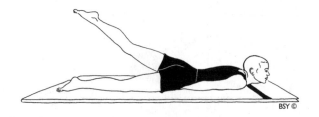

Ardha Shalabhasana (half locust pose)

Lie flat on the stomach with the hands under the thighs, palms downwards or hands clenched.

Keep both legs straight throughout the practice.

Place the chin on the floor.

Using the back muscles, raise the left leg as high as possible, keeping the other leg straight on the floor.

Retain the position for as long as possible without strain.

Lower the leg to the floor.

Repeat the same movement with the right leg.

This is one round.

Breathing: Inhale in the starting position.

Retain the breath inside while raising the leg and in the final position.

Exhale while lowering the leg to the starting position.

Duration: 3 to 5 rounds

Practice note: The left leg should be raised first so that pressure is applied to the right side of the abdomen to massage the ascending colon of the large intestine, following the direction of intestinal peristalsis.

Shalabhasana (locust pose)

Lie flat on the stomach with the legs and feet together and the soles of the feet uppermost.

The arms may be under the body or by the sides, with palms down or hands clenched.

This is the starting position.

Slowly raise the legs as high as possible, keeping them straight and together.

237

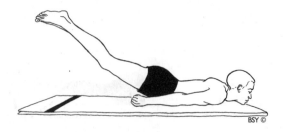

Hold the final position for as long as is comfortable without strain.
Slowly lower the legs to the floor.
This is one round.
Return to the starting position and relax the body with the head turned to one side.

Breathing: Inhale deeply in the starting position.
Retain the breath inside while raising the legs and holding the position. Exhale while lowering the legs.
Beginners may find it helpful to inhale while raising the legs.

Duration: 3 to 5 rounds.

Contra-indications: This asana requires a great deal of physical effort so it should no be practised by people with a weak heart, coronary thrombosis or high blood pressure. Those suffering from peptic ulcer, hernia, intestinal tuberculosis etc. should not practise shalabhasana.

Dhanurasana (bow pose)

Lie flat on the stomach with the legs and feet together, and the arms and hands beside the body.
Bend the knees and bring the heels close to the buttocks.
Clasp the hands around the ankles.
Place the chin on the floor.
This is the starting position.
Using the leg muscles and keeping the arms straight, push the feet away from the body.
Arch the neck and back, lifting the thighs, chest and head together.

238

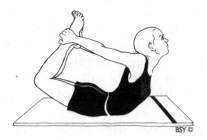

Hold the final position for as long as is comfortable and then, slowly lower the legs, chest and head to the starting position.

Release the starting position and relax until the respiration returns to normal. This is one round.

Breathing: Inhale deeply in the starting position.

Retain the breath while raising the body.

Retain the breath inside in the final position.

Exhale while returning to the prone position.

Duration: 3 to 5 rounds.

Contra-indications: People who suffer from a weak heart, high blood pressure, hernia, colitis, peptic or duodenal ulcers should not attempt this practice.

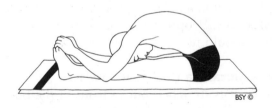

Paschimottanasana (back stretching pose)

Sit on the floor with the legs outstretched, feet together and hands on the knees.

This is the starting position.

Slowly bend forward from the hips, sliding the hands down the legs. Try to grasp the big toes with the fingers and thumbs; or hold the heels, ankles or any part of the legs that can be reached comfortably.

Hold the position for a few seconds. Relax the back and leg muscles allowing them to gently stretch.

Keeping the legs straight and utilizing the arm muscles, not the back muscles, begin to bend the elbows and gently bring the trunk down towards the legs, maintaining a firm grip on the toes, feet or legs.

Try to touch the knees with the forehead.

Do not strain.

This is the final position.

Hold the position for as long as is comfortable and relax.

Slowly return to the starting position.

This is one round.

Breathing: Inhale in the starting position.

Exhale slowly while bending forward.

Inhale in the static position.

Exhale while bringing the trunk further towards the legs with the arms.

Breathe slowly and deeply in the final position or retain the breath out if holding for a short duration.

Inhale while returning to the starting position.

Duration: Beginners may perform up to 5 rounds, remaining in the final position for only a short length of time. Adepts may maintain the final position for up to 5 minutes.

Contra-indications: People who suffer from slipped disc or sciatica should not practise this asana.

Ardha Matsyendrasana (half spinal twist)

Sit with the legs stretched out in front of the body.

Bend the right leg and place the right foot flat on the floor on the outside of the left knee.

Bend the left leg and bring the foot around to the right buttock.

Pass the left arm through the space between the chest and the right knee, and place it against the outside of the right leg.

Hold the right foot or ankle with the left hand, so that the right knee is close to the left armpit.

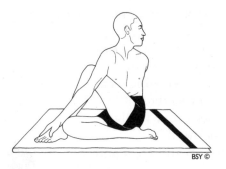

Sit up as straight as possible.

Slowly twist to the right. Use the left arm as a lever against the right leg to twist the trunk as far as possible without using the back muscles.

Look over the right shoulder keeping the head level.

Bend the right elbow and place the arm around the back of the left side of the waist.

Breathing: Inhale in the forward position.

Exhale while twisting the trunk.

Breathe deeply and slowly without strain in the final position. Inhale while returning to the starting position.

Duration: Practise once on each side, gradually increasing the holding time to 1 or 2 minutes on each side of the body or up to 30 breaths.

Contra-indications: People suffering from peptic ulcer, hernia or hyperthyroidism should only practise this pose under expert guidance.

People with sciatica or slipped disc may benefit from the variation of this asana, but great care should be taken.

Variation: For beginners and those with stiff bodies, the leg that is placed by the side of the buttock should remain straight and the hand holding the ankle may be wrapped around the opposite thigh, hugging the knee to the chest.

Vipareeta Karani Asana (inverted pose)

Lie flat on the back with the legs and feet together, arms by the side palms down.

Raise both legs, keeping them straight and together.

Move the legs over the body towards the head.

Push down on the arms and hands, raising the buttocks. Roll the spine off the floor, taking the legs further over the head.

Turn the palms up, bend the elbows and let the top of the

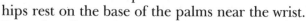

hips rest on the base of the palms near the wrist.

Keep the elbows close together.

Raise both the legs to the vertical position and relax the feet. In the final position, the trunk is at a 45 degree angle to the floor.

Close the eyes and relax in the final pose for as long as is comfortable.

To return to the starting position, lower the legs over the head, then place the hands on the floor, palms down.

Slowly lower the spine, vertebra by vertebra, along the floor.

When the buttocks reach the floor, lower the legs, keeping them straight.

Relax the body in shavasana.

Breathing: Inhale while in the lying position.

Retain the breath inside while assuming the final pose.

Once the body is steady in the final pose, practise normal or ujjayi breathing.

Retain the breath inside while lowering the body to the floor.

Duration: Beginners should practise for a few seconds only, gradually increasing the time over a period of weeks to an optimum of 3 to 5 minutes. This practice should be performed only once during the asana program.

Contra-indications: As for sarvangasana.

Sarvangasana (shoulder stand pose)

Lie on the back on a folded blanket.

Place the hands beside the body palms down.

With the support of the arms, slowly raise the legs to the vertical position, keeping them straight.

Press the arms and hands down on the floor. Slowly and smoothly roll the buttocks and spine off the floor, raising the trunk to a vertical position.

Place the hands behind the ribcage, slightly away from the spine.

Gently push the chest forward so that it presses firmly against the chin.

In the final position, the legs are vertical, together and in a straight line with the trunk.

Close the eyes. Relax the whole body in the final pose for as long as is comfortable.

To return to the starting position, bring the legs forward until the feet are above and behind the back of the head. Keep the legs straight.

Release the position of the hands and place the arms on the floor, palms down.

Gradually lower the spine to the floor, followed by the buttocks, until the legs resume their initial vertical position. Slowly lower the legs to the floor.

Relax in shavasana until the respiration and heartbeat return to normal.

243

Breathing: Inhale in the starting position.

Retain the breath inside while assuming the final pose.

Practise slow, deep abdominal breathing in the final pose when the body is steady.

Retain the breath inside while lowering the body to the floor.

Duration: As for vipareeta karani asana.

Contra-indications: This asana should not be practised by people suffering from enlarged thyroid, liver or spleen, cervical spondylitis, slipped disc, high blood pressure or other heart ailments, weak blood vessels in the eyes, thrombosis or impure blood. It should be avoided during menstruation and advanced stages of pregnancy.

29

Pranayama

Pranayama is a series of techniques that aim at stimulating and increasing the vital energy in the body by directing it to particular areas for special purposes, including healing. Pranayama ensures that the flow of vital energy in the body is free and unimpeded, helping to maintain good health.

Pranayama, correctly performed, forms the bridge between body and mind. It should be performed gently and with awareness. It should never be forced in the expectation of better results, as this is a block to success. It is better to practise below your maximum capacity at first so that you do not suffer strain.

The following points should be carefully read and carried out before starting to do pranayama:

- The bladder, stomach and intestines should be empty. Wait for at least four hours after meals.
- Do pranayama after asana but before meditation practices.
- During pranayama there should be no strain. Breath retention must not be done for longer than is comfortable. This is most important as the lungs are very delicate organs and any misuse can lead to injury.
- Practise in a well ventilated (not windy), clean and pleasant environment.
- Pranayama should not be practised during illness, although simple techniques such as breath awareness and abdominal breathing in shavasana may be performed.

Always consult a yoga therapist or teacher before using any pranayama for therapeutic purposes.

• All pranayama practices should be performed in a comfortable sitting position, preferably sukhasana (easy pose), padmasana (lotus pose), siddha yoni asana (accomplished pose for women) or siddhasana (accomplished pose for men). The back should be straight, the head upright and the eyes closed. Before commencing any practice you should prepare your body and mind to ensure that any areas of tension are relaxed.

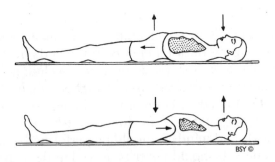

Abdominal (or diaphragmatic) breathing

Lie in shavasana and relax the whole body.

Observe the spontaneous breath without controlling it in any way. Continue observing the natural breath for some time.

Place the right hand on the abdomen just above the navel and the left hand on the centre of the chest.

Slowly inhale and expand the abdomen as much as possible.

Slowly exhale while contracting the abdomen.

Try not to move the chest or shoulders.

The right hand moves up with inhalation and down with exhalation.

The left hand should not move with the breath.

Continue breathing slowly and deeply.

At the end of the inhalation the navel will be at its highest point.

On exhalation the navel moves downward towards the spine.

Continue for a few minutes.

Yogic breathing

Sit in a meditation posture or lie in shavasana and relax the whole body.

Inhale slowly and deeply, allowing the abdomen to expand fully.

At the end of abdominal expansion, as the inhalation continues start to expand the chest outward and upward. When the ribs are fully expanded, inhale a little more until expansion is felt in the clavicular area, the upper portion of the lungs around the base of the neck.

This completes one inhalation.

The whole process should be one continuous movement. Now start to exhale.

First, relax the clavicular area in the upper part of the chest; then allow the chest to contract downward and then inward.

Next, the abdomen contracts as the diaphragm pushes upward and toward the lungs.

Without straining, empty the lungs by drawing the abdominal wall toward the spine.

The entire breath movement should be harmonious and flowing.

Hold the breath for a few seconds at the end of exhalation.

This completes one round of yogic breathing.

At first perform 5 to 10 rounds and slowly increase to 10 minutes daily.

Practice note: Once control of the breathing process has been established, the clavicular technique is dropped and yogic breathing is modified to become a combination of abdominal and thoracic breathing.

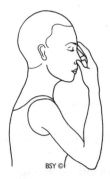

Nadi Shodhana Pranayama (psychic network purification)
Hand position: Nasagra Mudra (nosetip position)

Rest the index and middle fingers of the right hand on the eyebrow centre.

The thumb is above the right nostril and the ring finger above the left.

These two fingers control the flow of breath in the nostrils by alternately pressing on one nostril, blocking the flow of breath, and then the other.

Technique 1: Preparatory practice

Sit in any comfortable meditation posture. Keep the head and spine upright.

Relax the whole body and close the eyes. Practise yogic breathing.

Adopt nasagra mudra with the right hand and place the left hand on the knee.

Close the right nostril with the thumb.

Inhale and exhale through the left nostril 5 times. The breath should be absoultely silent

The rate of inhalation/exhalation should be normal.

After 5 breaths release the pressure of the thumb on the right nostril and close the left nostril with the ring finger. Inhale and exhale through the right nostril 5 times, keeping the respiration rate normal.

Lower the hand and breathe 5 times through both nostrils together.

This is one round.

Practise 5 rounds or for 3 to 5 minutes, making sure that there is no sound as the air passes through the nostrils. After practising for 15 days go on to technique 2.

Technique 2: Alternate nostril breathing

In this technique the duration of inhalation/exhalation is controlled.

Close the right nostril with the thumb and breathe in using yogic breathing through the left nostril.

At the same time count mentally, "1, Om; 2, Om; 3, Om", until the inhalation ends comfortably. This is the basic count.

Close the left nostril with the ring finger, release the pressure of the thumb on the right nostril and breathe out through the right nostril, making the same count. The time for inhalation and exhalation should be equal, a ratio of 1:1.

Next, inhale through the right nostril, keeping the same count.

At the end of inhalation close the right nostril, open the left nostril and exhale through the left nostril, counting as before.

This is one round.

Practise 5 to 10 rounds.

Ratio and timing: After a few days, if there is no difficulty, increase the length of inhalation/exhalation by one count keeping the same ratio. Continue in this way, increasing the inhalation/exhalation by one count as it becomes easy.

After perfecting the above ratio, it may be changed to 1:2.

Sheetkari (hissing breath)

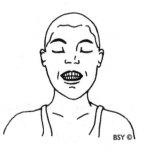

Have the teeth lightly together and the lips apart.

The tongue may be flat of folded in khechari mudra.

Breathe in slowly and deeply through the teeth.

Close the mouth and breathe out slowly through the nose. This is one round. Practise 9 rounds.

Contra-indications: Not to be practised by people with low blood pressure or respiratory disorders such as asthma and bronchitis. Those with heart disease should practise without breath retention. Sufferers of chronic constipation should avoid sheetkari.

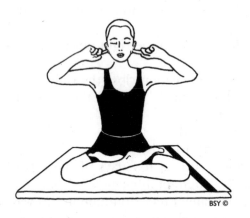

Bhramari Pranayama (humming bee breath)

Sit in a comfortable meditation asana with the hands resting on the knees.

The lips should remain gently closed with the jaw relaxed and the teeth slightly separated.

Raise the arms sideways, bringing the hands to the ears. Use the index or middle finger to plug the ears.

Breathe in through the nose.

Exhale slowly while making a deep, steady humming sound like that of the black bee.

The humming sound should be smooth, even and continuous for the duration of the exhalation.

This is one round.

At the end of exhalation, breathe in deeply and repeat the process.

Perform 5 rounds.

Duration: Practise 5 to 10 rounds in the beginning, then slowly increase to 10 to 15 minutes.

Contra-indications: Bhramari should not be performed while lying down, or by those with severe ear infections.

Ujjayi Pranayama (the psychic breath)

Close the eyes and relax the whole body.

Try to feel or imagine that the breath is being drawn in and out through the throat, not through the nostrils.

Gently contract the glottis so that a soft snoring sound like the breathing of a sleeping baby is produced.

Practise abdominal breathing.

Both inhalation and exhalation should be long and even and at the same time relaxed.

The sound of the breath should be just be audible to the practitioner.

When this has been mastered, the tongue can be folded back into khechari mudra, so that the lower surface lies in contact with the upper palate.

Duration: Practise for 10 to 20 minutes.

Contra-indications: People who are very introverted by nature should not perform this practice.

Practice note: Ujjayi may be performed in any position, standing, sitting or lying, except when practised with khechari mudra, which should be done in a sitting position.

Bhastrika Pranayama (bellows breath)
Technique 1: Preparatory practice

Sit in any comfortable meditation posture with the hands on the knees.

Keep the head and spine straight, close the eyes and relax the whole body.

Take a deep breath in and breathe out forcefully through the nose. Do not strain.

Immediately afterwards breathe in with the same force.

During inhalation the abdomen moves outward and during exhalation the abdomen moves inward.

Continue in this manner, counting 10 breaths.

At the end of 10 breaths take a deep breath in and breathe out slowly.

This is one round.

Practise up to 5 rounds.

Practice note: When accustomed to this breathing, gradually increase the speed, always keeping the breath rhythmical.

Inhalation and exhalation must be equal in force and duration.

Technique 2: Left, right and both nostrils

Raise the right hand and perform nasagra mudra.

Left nostril: Close the right nostril with the thumb.

Breathe in and out forcefully, without straining, through the left nostril 10 times. Count each breath mentally. The abdomen should expand and contract rhythmically with the breath in a pumping action.

Do not expand the chest or raise the shoulders. The body should not jerk.

After 10 respirations, breathe in deeply through the left nostril keeping the right nostril closed.

Close both nostrils and hold the breath inside for a few seconds. Exhale through the left nostril.

Right nostril: Close the left nostril and perform the same practice in the same way in the right nostril.

After 10 respirations, breathe in deeply through the right nostril keeping the left nostril closed.

Close both nostrils and hold the breath inside for a few seconds.

Exhale through the right nostril.

Both nostrils: Open both nostrils bringing the right hand to the knee and perform the same practice in the same way through both nostrils.

After 10 respirations, breathe in deeply through both nostrils.

Close both nostrils and hold the breath inside for a few seconds.

Exhale through both nostrils.

Breathing through the left, the right and both nostrils, as above, forms one complete round.

Practise 3 to 5 rounds.

Breathing: Bhastrika may be practised at three different breath rates: slow (one breath every two seconds), medium (one breath every second) and fast (two breaths per second), depending on the capacity of the practitioner. Beginners are advised to start with the slow rate until proficient, then increase the rate.

The number of breaths may be increased by 5 per month to a maximum of 40 to 50 through the left, right and both nostrils.

Duration: Up to 5 rounds. Slowly increase the duration of retention up to 30 seconds. Do not strain.

Contra-indications: Bhastrika should not be practised by people suffering from high blood pressure, heart disease, hernia, gastric ulcer, stroke, epilepsy or vertigo. Those with lung diseases such as asthma and chronic bronchitis should practise only under expert guidance.

30

Mudra and Bandha

Mudras are a combination of subtle physical movements which alter mood, attitude and perception, and which deepen awareness and concentration. A mudra may involve the whole body in a combination of asana, pranayama, bandha and visualisation techniques or it may be a simple hand position.

Bandhas are the physical techniques that allow the practitioner to control the different organs and nerves of the body, and they constitute a very important group of practices. During the performance of bandhas various parts of the body are contracted or tightened, massaging the internal organs and their nerves and blood vessels.

Ashwini Mudra (horse gesture)
Sit in a comfortable meditation pose.

Contract the sphincter muscles of the anus for a few seconds without straining, then relax them for a few seconds.

Repeat the practice for as long as is comfortable.

Contraction and relaxation should be smooth and rhythmic.

You can also inhale while contracting and exhale while relaxing.

Contra-indications: Not to be practised by people with anal fistula.

Bhujangini Mudra (cobra respiration)

Sit in a comfortable meditative pose. Close the eyes and relax the body, particularly the abdomen.

Try to suck in air through the mouth and draw it into the stomach, not the lungs, in a series of gulps as though drinking water.

Expand the stomach as much as possible.

Hold the air for a short time and then expel it by belching.

Duration: 3 to 5 times is sufficient for general purposes.

Khechari Mudra (tongue lock)

Sit in any comfortable meditation pose.

Fold the tongue back so that the lower surface touches the upper soft palate.

Perform ujjayi pranayama. Breathe slowly and deeply.

Hold for as long as is comfortable.

Beginners can relax the tongue for a few seconds, then resume the practice.

Duration: Practise for 5 to 10 minutes.

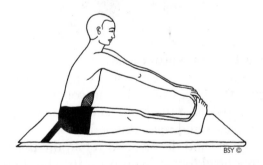

Tadagi Mudra (barrelled abdomen technique)

Sit with the legs outstretched, feet slightly apart.

Place the hands on the knees, keeping the head and spine straight.

Lean forward and grasp the big toes with the thumbs, index and second fingers, keeping the head facing forward.

Inhale slowly and deeply, expanding the abdominal muscles to their fullest extent.

Retain the breath inside for a comfortable length of time without straining.

Exhale slowly and deeply while relaxing the abdomen.

Maintain the hold on the toes.

Repeat the breathing up to 10 times.

Then release the toes and return to the starting position. This is 1 round.

Duration: Practise 3 to 5 rounds.

Contra-indications: Pregnant women and those suffering from hernia or prolapse should avoid this practice.

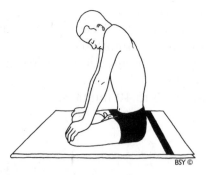

Jalandhara Bandha (throat lock)

Sit in siddha/siddha yoni asana with the head and spine straight. The knees should be in contact with the floor.

Place the palms of the hands on the knees.

Close the eyes and relax the body.

Inhale slowly and deeply, and retain the breath inside.

Bend the head forward and press the chin tightly against the chest.

Straighten the arms, pressing the knees down with the hands.

Hunch the shoulders upward and forward.

Stay in the final position for as long as the breath can be held comfortably.

Do not strain.

Relax the shoulders, bend the arms and slowly release the lock, raise the head and then exhale.

Repeat when the respiration has returned to normal.

Contra-indications: People suffering from cervical spondylosis, high intracranial pressure, vertigo, high blood pressure or heart disease should not do this practice.

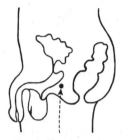 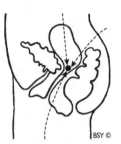

Fig. 1: For the male   Fig. 2: For the female

Moola Bandha (perineal contraction)

Sit in a meditative pose, preferably siddhasana/siddha yoni asana.

Close the eyes and relax the whole body.

Mentally locate a point halfway between the anus and genital organs in the male and at the cervix in the female.

Slowly inhale and contract this point upward without moving either the anus or the genitals. Retain the position for as long as is comfortable, then exhale and release.

Repeat up to 10 times.

Precaution: This practice should only be performed under the guidance of an experienced yoga teacher.

Uddiyana Bandha (abdominal contraction)

Sit in a meditative pose, preferably siddhasana/siddha yoni asana.

Place the palms of the hands flat on the knees.

Close the eyes and relax the whole body.

Breathe in deeply through the nostrils and exhale, emptying the lungs as much as possible.

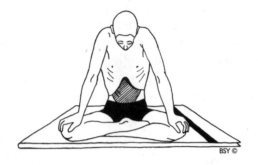

Lean forward and press down on the knees with the palms.

Straighten the elbows and raise the shoulders.

Press the chin against the chest.

Contract the abdominal muscles inward and upward.

Hold the abdominal lock and the breath outside for as long as possible without straining.

Release the abdominal lock, bend the elbows and lower the shoulders.

Raise the head and slowly inhale.

Allow the respiration to return to normal.

Breathing: Uddiyana bandha is performed with external retention only.

Duration: 3 rounds in the beginning, gradually increasing to 10 rounds over a few months.

Precaution: This is an advanced technique and should be attempted only under guidance.

Contra-indications: People suffering from colitis, stomach or intestinal ulcer, diaphragmatic hernia, glaucoma and raised intracranial pressure should not perform this practice. It should be avoided by pregnant women.

31

Meditative Practices

Meditative practices are important for achieving deep states of relaxation and inner awareness. When this is achieved we reach the subconscious and unconscious problems that plague our lives and become able to remove the root factors responsible for most digestive disorders.

Yoga Nidra (psychic sleep)
Yoga nidra is a state of inner awareness combined with complete relaxation. Though the body may sleep the mind is totally aware and awake.

Preparation: Lie in shavasana and adjust your physical body so that you are comfortable. Close your eyes and do not open them until the practice is over. Follow all instructions mentally and make yourself free from all intellectualization. Two important points to remember are: no physical movement of any kind and no sleeping. You have to keep awake throughout.
Develop awareness of your whole physical body from top to bottom. Complete awareness of the whole physical body.
Complete awareness of the whole body.
Rotation of consciousness: Prepare for rotation of consciousness through the different centres of the body. Repeat the name of a particular organ or part of the body in your

mind and try to develop awareness of it for just a moment. Let the consciousness flow. For instance, if I say 'right hand thumb', you have to say mentally 'right hand thumb', without moving it, and then go on. I will lead your consciousness to the different parts of the body. Just keep yourself very alert and develop awareness.

Right side: Say mentally: right hand thumb, little finger, index finger, middle finger, ring finger, little finger, palm, wrist, forearm, elbow, upper arm, shoulder, armpit, right side of the chest, waist, hip, thigh, knee, calf muscle, ankle, heel, sole, the right toes, one, two, three, four, five.

Left side: Go to the left side of the body: left hand thumb, index finger, middle finger, ring finger, little finger, palm, wrist, forearm, elbow, upper arm, shoulder, armpit, left side of the chest, waist, hip, thigh, knee, calf muscle, ankle, heel, sole, the left toes, one, two, three, four, five.

Back: Go to the back side, to the back of the body. Take your mind to the back of the head which is touching the ground, right shoulder blade, left shoulder blade, right buttock, left buttock, right side of the back, left side of the back, whole spinal cord.

Front: Go to the top of the head, the crown of the head, the forehead, right temple, left temple, right eyebrow, left eyebrow, centre of the eyebrows, right eye, left eye, right nostril, right cheek, left cheek, right ear, left ear, upper lip, lower lip, teeth, gums, tongue, lower jaw, throat, right side of the chest, left side of the chest, centre of the chest, upper abdomen, navel centre, right pelvis, left pelvis.

Digestive tract: Now take your awareness to the digestive tract. As you follow the instructions you are sending prana to each and every part. As you pass by you direct prana with your awareness and with your thought power. Starting from the mouth, feel as though you are moving back into the throat and oesophagus, running from the mouth down to the stomach at the bottom of the left chest. On the right side of the stomach, under the right side of the ribcage and diaphragm, is the liver, the biggest organ in the body. Behind the stomach, next to the spinal column and in the centre of the body, is the pancreas. Move the awareness to the small intestines which lead from the stomach and fill most of the central portion of the abdomen. In the right groin the small intestine joins the large intestine which ascends to just under the right rib cage, moves across the abdomen to the bottom of the left rib cage and then descends to the pelvis. It centralizes at the level of the left groin and ends at the rectum and anus.

Move back to the mouth and once more become aware of the complete digestive tract. Let your awareness move throughout the length of the body, and try to feel into the different organs. As you move through, you should feel that you are simultaneously sending prana and consciousness together.

Now become aware of the whole digestive tract simultaneously, complete awareness of the digestive tract simultaneously, complete awareness of the digestive system. I am awake, I am not sleeping, I am awake and aware of the instructions being given.

Breath awareness: Develop awareness of the normal breath in the abdomen. Do not alter the breath but be aware that it is moving and that it continues to do so 15 times every minute or 21,600 times a day. Be aware of the rise and fall of the abdomen. With every inhalation it rises and with every exhalation it falls. Just be aware of this flowing, wave-like motion for a few moments.

Feel that with every inhalation you are taking in life, giving prana, warm and golden, tingling energy. With every exhalation you are throwing out the impurities of the body and mind, the toxins, tensions, worries, frustrations, anger, resentment and guilt. With every exhalation you become more and more relaxed.

Go on in this way for 5 to 10 minutes, becoming more and more relaxed with each breath you take.

261

Visualization: Visualize the internal organs of the body. Try to remember the illustration at the end of this book. Try to visualize in your mind's eye the digestive tract from mouth to anus. Bring into sharp and clear focus the different components. Mouth, throat, oesophagus, stomach, liver, pancreas, small intestine, large intestine, rectum, anus. Bring each part into focus so that every detail becomes clear to you. Let the organs come by themselves. After some time you will see the individual cells contributing their own special function to the maintenance of total integrity and the higher and larger function.

As each part becomes clear in your mind, visualize the tract being flooded with prana. The prana is a golden coloured light which is sparkling and shining, and flows along the tract from mouth to anus.

As prana passes each organ, it imbues that part with vitality and health. You can actually see the digestive system filled with this light, life-giving force permeating through into the very heart of each organ and cell, leaving it with a golden colour. You can see the function improve. The digestive tract takes on a much brighter and sharper aura, as though the structure itself has actually been altered.

Go on examining the different aspects of structure and function in the digestive tract. Try to see how the energies that are inherent work within. How do they fit together? How do they contribute to the whole of the body's health, vitality and longevity? Now take your awareness to the breath, the rhythmic and natural breath in the nose, throat, chest, abdomen. How does the breath link up with the digestion?

Finish: Take your awareness to the physical body. Move your fingers and toes and stretch the body, rolling it from side to side. When you are ready, keeping the eyes closed, sit up in a comfortable sitting position and open the eyes.

Hari Om Tat Sat

Antar Mouna (inner silence)

In this practice we become aware of the inner world. Though we practise for a short period each day, this practice extends into our every waking moment and can be practised for 24 hours a day, anywhere, at any time. It is purely and simply the cultivation of internal awareness of thoughts, emotional reactions and so on, so that we clearly perceive our reactions to life's situations and thereby we can speed up our personal evolution.

There are six stages to the practice but of these only two concern us here: the cultivation of awareness of outside sounds and occurrences happening around you; to be followed by the withdrawal of your awareness from all outside stimuli, so as to become aware of the workings of the mind. The other stages are really the outgrowth of the first two and come only after practice has been cultivated.

Stage 1: Awareness of external stimuli

In the first stage we become aware of external sounds and sensations. Do not fight with your mind, do not struggle with the sense perceptions, but become aware or become a spectator of them. Just allow awareness to grow so that the mind and senses are trained to become undisturbed by sensual experiences. Neither sound, sight, taste, touch, smell, nor anything else should disturb you. The senses are calmed by the attitude of 'I am the seer of experiences'. Be an observer, a witness of the interaction between sound and the ears, sight and eyes, and so on.

This stage can be practised anywhere, at home, in the car, amongst friends, while eating, any time of day or night, not only in the midst of calmness and silence. In this way we develop the attitude of a calm and silent witness.

Stage 2: Awareness of spontaneous thought process

Stage 2 means withdrawal of awareness from the outside into the mind, the thinking process, the awareness of the spontaneous thoughts that come and go of their own

263

accord. You must remain a silent witness of every thought that is going on in your mind. You will find thoughts coming up, unstimulated, unagitated, from the very depth of your past. Meaningless, insignificant, in the form of a glimpse, in the twinkling of an eye.

Unless you are a careful witness, it will not be possible for you to follow the swift speed of your consciousness.

Sometimes there is a mental block and no thoughts come. It means that the consciousness is not manifesting itself. The mind goes on thinking, but you do not see it. There is a veil over the thought process; tear it off and find thought after thought.

When a thought comes, see it and register it in your mind. There are many thoughts, some of which you do not wish to register and also some from which you may even want to escape.

It is natural for our psychological nature to suppress things. If the veil is removed the mind can manifest itself and when it works in freedom there is joy and happiness. If the past expresses itself while you are practising being a detached witness, you become free from agony and reactions. During this practice make sure to:

i) Allow yourself freedom

ii) See yourself

Don't oppose any thought, don't hesitate, don't suffer from any thought of guilt.

Free thinking but vigilant seeing. You are not the thought, but you are the witness of the thought. Absolute detachment. You will have to try it. Don't associate yourself with any thought, keep yourself separate, as a seer of thought, as a beholder of experiences. You are not the thought. You are not the energy of your consciousness, you do not hate any thought and you do not love any thought, you do not like any thought and you do not dislike any thought, but allow them to manifest. It is difficult to think consciously, the thinking process is spontaneous.

Withdraw the curtain of inhibition so that the thoughts are allowed to come to the surface spontaneously. When the consciousness manifests itself freely, when the curtains of inhibition are fully or partially withdrawn, then the first horrible thoughts will come. Good thoughts will come later. Remember that it does not matter which thoughts are manifesting, good or bad, just be a witness. As though you are watching a television set or a movie, or a passing train. The thoughts come and go like the waters of a river.

Don't be shy; don't be agonized; remain a witness to the whole process. Continuous, unbroken awareness. The inner consciousness must be constantly vigilant, watching peace, disturbance, agitation, desirable and undesirable thoughts. Inside and outside, one must watch all feelings, all the thoughts, all the dimensions of consciousness.

Now bring your mind back to the physical body as the practice of antar mouna comes to an end.

Hari Om Tat Sat

Ajapa Japa (spontaneous repetition of mantra)

The constant repetition of a mantra is known as japa. Japa becomes ajapa (spontaneous) japa when the mantra automatically repeats itself without conscious effort.

Sitting in a comfortable meditative posture, keep the back straight and close the eyes. Have the hands on the knees in jnana or chin mudra. After preparing the body and mind for the practice, begin ujjayi pranayama with khechari mudra.

Go on with ujjayi for a few minutes until you become established in the practice. Then become aware of the frontal passage. This psychic passage extends from the navel to the throat, and should initially be imagined as a thin, thread-like passage with a golden colour until the passage becomes a part of your consciousness.

265

You should imagine the breath is ascending and descending the frontal passage. With each breath in, the breath rises from the navel to the throat, and with each breath out it falls from the throat to the navel. The breath and consciousness rise and fall together in the frontal passage. Now add the mantra *So ham* to the breath. *So* rises with the inhalation and *ham* descends with exhalation.

Go on for some time, awareness of the rise and fall of the breath, synchronized with the mantra. When this preliminary practice is easy for you, take the awareness to the spinal passage, sushumna, and move the breath and the mantra from mooladhara to ajna on inhalation, and from ajna to mooladhara on exhalation. Move the breath in the spinal cord for as long as is comfortable, 49 rounds, or at least 10 minutes.

Then stop the mantra, release khechari and become aware of the natural breath in the nostrils. Become aware of the physical body and the external environment.

Hari Om Tat Sat

Chidakasha Dharana (viewing the space of consciousness)

Chidakasha is the space of consciousness located in the area of the head. If you close your eyes for a few seconds you will see a space in front. This is the mind screen on which you can view many subtle visions and impressions manifesting from the deeper levels of your consciousness.

Sit in a comfortable meditative posture, with the back straight, eyes closed and the hands in chin or jnana mudra.

Relax all the tension in your body and mind and make your body perfectly still and steady. There should be no physical movement of any kind, as the steadier the body is, the steadier is the mind.

Become aware of the breath. It is an automatic process, just watch it.

After a few minutes draw your awareness to chidakasha, the space in front of the closed eyes. Withdraw your mind and concentrate on the forehead from inside, as though you are looking at a wall. You will become aware of a space or sky, the inner space or the inner sky which is known as chidakasha.

The awareness should be relaxed awareness. Do not strain your body or your eyes to try to see anything. Let the experiences come by themselves. Allow everything to happen slowly, spontaneously and naturally.

Try to see the roof, floor and walls of this space in front of the closed eyes. Any visions that come should be observed with the attitude of a detached witness, an impartial observer, as you learned in antar mouna.

Now chant *Om* three times.

Hari Om Tat Sat

Appendices

Appendix A

Internal Organs

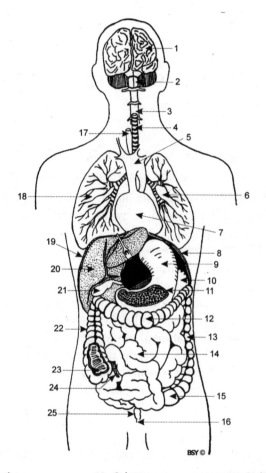

1. Brain	10. Spleen	18. Right Lung
2. Cerebellum	11. Pancreas	19. Diaphragm
3. Spinal cord	12. Transverse colon	20. Liver
4. Trachea	(large intestine)	21. Gall Bladder
5. Aorta	13. Descending colon	22. Ascending colon
6. Left Lung	14. Small intestine	23. Cecum
7. Heart	15. Sigmoid colon	24. Appendix
8. Diaphragm	16. Anus	25. Rectum
9. Stomach	17. Oesophagus	

Appendix B

Sutras on Digestion

अन्नाद्वै प्रजा: प्रजायन्ते । या: काश्च पृथिवीःश्रिता: । अथो अन्नेनैव जीवन्ति।
अथैनदपि यन्त्यन्तत: । अन्नं हि भूतानां ज्येष्ठम् । तस्मात्सर्वौषधमुच्यते ।
सर्वं वै तेऽन्नमाप्नुवन्ति । येऽन्नं ब्रह्मोपासते । अन्नं हि भूतानां ज्येष्ठम् ।
तस्मात्सर्वौषध-मुच्यते । अन्नाद् भूतानि जायन्ते। जातान्यन्नेन वर्धन्ते । अद्यतेऽत्ति
च भूतानि । तस्मादन्नं तदुच्यत इति ॥ १ ॥

Whatsoever living beings live on this earth, truly they are born from
food, also they remain alive on food alone and in the same way they
return to it at the end. Food is, verily, the first among all that is
created, therefore it is said to be the medicine for all. One who
meditates on food as Brahman, surely obtains all food. Verily, food
is the first among all, hence it is the universal remedy. All creatures
are born from food, they grow up by food. All beings consume it and
are consumed by it, hence it is regarded as food.

Taittiriya Upanishad (2:1)

इष्टवर्णगन्धरसस्पर्शं विधिविहितमन्त्रपानं प्राणिनां प्राणिसंज्ञकानां प्राणमाचक्षते
कुशला:, प्रत्यक्षफलदर्शनात्; तदिन्धना ह्यन्तरग्ने: स्थिति:, तत् सत्त्वमूर्जयति,
तच्छ-रीरधातुव्यूहबलवर्णेन्द्रियप्रसादकरं यथोक्तमुपसेव्यमानं, विपरीतमहिताय
संपद्यते ॥ ३ ॥

Such diets and drinks whose colour, smell, taste and touch are
pleasing to the senses and conducive to the health, if taken in

272

accordance with the rules, in fact, represent the very life of living beings. The effect of using such diets and drinks can be perceived directly. If consumed according to rules, they provide fuel for the fire of digestion, promote mental as well as physical strength, strength of tissue elements and complexion and they are pleasing to the senses. Otherwise they are harmful.

Charaka Samhita (27:3)

हिताभिर्जुह्‌याञ्नित्यमन्तरग्निं समाहितः। अन्नपानसमिद्धिर्ना मात्राकालौ विचारयन् ॥ ३४५ ॥ आहिताग्निः सदा पथ्यान्यन्तरग्नौ जुहोति यः। दिवसे दिवसे ब्रह्म जपत्यथ ददाति च ॥ ३४६ ॥ नरं निःश्रेयसे युक्तं सात्म्यज्ञं पानभोजने। भजन्ते नामयाः केचिद्द्राविनोऽप्यन्तरादृते ॥ ३४७ ॥

Paying due consideration to the quantity and time, a self-controlled man should regularly take such useful food and drinks as are conducive to the internal power of digestion including metabolism. Like an *ahitagni* (one who performs yajna) one who takes a diet conducive to the power of digestion, being aware of the wholesomeness of food and drink, who resorts to meditation on Brahma and charity, enjoys bliss without any disease during the present as well as future lives.

Charaka Samhita (27:345–347)

प्राणाः प्राणभृतामन्नमन्त्रं लोकोऽभिधावति। वर्णः प्रसादः सौस्वर्यं जीवितं प्रतिभा सुखम् ॥ तुष्टिः पुष्टिर्बलं मेधा सर्वमन्ने प्रतिष्ठितम्। लौकिकं कर्म यद्-वृत्तौ स्वगतौ यच्च वदिकम् ॥

Food sustains the life of living beings. All living beings in the universe require food. Complexion, clarity, good voice, longevity, genius, happiness, satisfaction, nourishment, strength and intellect are all conditioned by food. Professional activities leading to happiness in this world, vedic rituals leading to the abode in heaven and observance of truth, brahmacharya leading to salvation, all are based on food.

Charaka Samhita (27:349–350)

The man who stops just a little before he feels he has had enough retains the joy of eating. The big eater invites diseases. Much pain is saved if one learns to eat only what has been found to suit one's own health and to say "No" so as to exercise self-restraint in respect to quantity. The ignorant man who eats beyond the power of his digestion (lit. 'the measure of the fire') must be prepared for all sorts of ailments.

Tiru Kurral

सुस्निग्धमधुराहारश्चतुर्थांशविवर्जितः । भुज्यते शिवसंप्रीत्यै मिताहारः स उच्यते ॥ ५८ ॥ कट्वम्लतीक्ष्णलवणोष्णहरीतशाक सौवीरतैलतिलसर्षप मद्यमत्स्यान् । आजादिमांसदधित्रकुलत्थकोलपिण्याकहिगुलशुनाद्यमपथ्यमाहुः ॥ ५९ ॥ भोजनमहितं विद्यात्पुनरस्योष्णीकृतं रूक्षम् । अतिलवणमम्लयुक्तं कदशनशाकोत्कटं वर्ज्यम् ॥ ६० ॥ गोधूमशालियवषाष्टिकशोभनान्नंक्षी-राज्यखण्डनवनीतसितामधूनि । शुंठीपटोलकफलादिकपंचशाकंमुद्गादि-दिव्यमुदकंच यमींद्रपथ्यम् ॥ ६२ ॥ पुष्टं सुमधुरं स्निग्धं गव्यं धातुप्रपोषणम् । मनोभिलषितं योग्यं योगी भोजनमाचरेत् ॥ ६३ ॥

Moderate diet means pleasant, sweet food, leaving one quarter of the stomach free. The act of eating is to be dedicated to Lord Shiva (the highest consciousness). The following are considered as being unwholesome: sour, pungent and hot foods, mustard, alcohol, fish, meat, curd, chick peas, fruit of the jujube, asafoetida and garlic. It is also advisable to avoid reheated foods, an excess of salt or acid foods that are hard to digest or are woody... The following items can be used without hesitation: wheat products, rice, milk, oils, sweets, honey, dried ginger, cucumber, vegetables and pure water. The yogi should eat nourishing foods, sweet and mixed with milk. They should benefit the senses and stimulate the various bodily functions.

Hatha Yoga Pradipika (I:58–60, 62, 66)

मिताहारं विनायस्तु योगारंभं तु कारयेत्। नानारोगो भवेत्तस्य किंचिद्योगो न सिद्ध्यति ॥ १६ ॥ कठिनं दुरितं पूर्तिमुष्णं पर्युषितं तथा। अतिशीतं चातिचोग्रं भक्ष्यं योगी विवर्जयेत् ॥ ३ ॥ प्रातः स्नानोपवासादि कायक्लेशविधिं तथा।

एकाहारं निराहारं यामान्ते च न कारयेत् ॥ ३१ ॥ एवं विधिविधानेन प्राणायामं समाचरेत् आरम्भे प्रथमे कुर्यात् क्षीराज्यं नित्यभोजनम्। मध्यान्हे चैव सायान्हे भोजनद्वयमाचरेत् ॥ ३२ ॥

He who practises yoga without moderation in diet incurs various diseases and obtains no success. A yogi should avoid hard (not easily digestible), sinful, or putrid, very hot, or very stale, as well as very cooling or very exciting food. He should avoid early (before sunrise) baths, fasting, etc., or anything giving pain to the body; so also is prohibited to him eating only once a day, or not eating at all. But he may remain without food for three hours. Regulating his life in this way, let him practise pranayama. In the beginning, before commencing it, he should take a little milk and ghee daily, and take his food twice daily, once at noon and once in the evening.

Gherand Samhita (5:16, 30–32)

References

Digestive Prana
[1] S. Freidman, *J. Nervous and Mental Diseases*, 166:110–116, 1978

Am I Hungry?
[1] E.F. Adolph, *Amer. J. Physiol.*, 151:110–125, 1947
[2] R.T. Bellows & W.P. van Wagenen, *Amer. J. Physiol.*, 126:13–19, 1939

Digestion and the Mind
[1] G.F. Mahl, 'Physiological Changes During Chronic Fear', *Annals of New York Academy of Science*, 56:240–252, 1952
[2] S. Wolf & H.G. Wolff, *Human Gastric Function*, London, Oxford Uni. Press, 1943
[3, 4, 5] 'Mind-Body Link', *Science News*, 108, Dec. 20–27, 1975

Pass the Antacid, Please
[1] H.W. Davenport, *Physiology of the Digestive Tract*, Year Book Medical Publishers, Chicago, 1968

What's Eating You?
[1] S. Wolf & H.G. Wolff, *Human Gastric Function* (2nd edn), Oxford Uni. Press, New York, 1947

Feeling Constipated?

[1] *J. Am. Med. Assoc*. 38:1304–5, 1902

[2] *Samson Wright's Applied Physiology* (11th edn), Oxford Uni. Press, London, 1965, p. 370

[3] H.W. Davenport, *Physiology of the Digestive System*, Year Book Medical Pub. Inc., Chicago, 1968, p. 217

Painful Piles

[1] P.H. Lord, *Proc. Roy. Soc. Med*., 61:935, 1968

Diarrhoea

[1] *Davidson's Principles and Practice of Medicine* (11th edn), ed. J. Macleod, Churchill Livingstone, London & New York, 1975

[2] H.W. Davenport, *Physiology of the Digestive Tract* (2nd edn), Year Book Med. Pub. Inc., Chicago, 1968, p.76

[3] Cecil-Loeb, *Textbook of Medicine* (11th edn), P.B. Beeson and W.M Dermott, Saunders Co., Philadelphia and London, 1963, p. 822

[4] D.H. Funkenstein, 'The Physiology of Fear and Anger', *Scientific American*, May 1955

Obesity

[1] J.L. Knittle & J. Hirsh, 'Effect of Early Nutrition in the Development of Rat Epididymal Fat Pads: Cellularity and Metabolism', *J. Clin. Invest*., 47:2091, 1968

[2] S. Schachter, 'Obesity and Eating: Internal and External Cues Differentially Affect the Eating   Behaviour of Obese and Normal Subjects' *Science*, 161:751, 1968

[3] *Dorland's Illustrated Medical Dictionary*, 25th edn, W.B. Saunders, Philadelphia-London-Toronto, 1974

Poor Nutrition

[1-7] R. Lewin, Starved Brains', *Psychology Today*, 9 (4), Sept. 1975

Diet and Disease

[1-3] P.B. Chowka, 'Cancer: Metaphor for Modern Times', *East West Journal*, 7 (3), March 1977

277

Index of Practices